Living with Mental Illness in a Globalised World

Living with Mental Illness in a Globalised World systematically examines the manifold contributions to the burdens of living with mental illness in a developing and globalised world. It explores the stigma of mental illness, the burden of which compares to the symptoms of and is sometimes considered more disabling than the illness itself.

The book starts by reviewing the socio-psychological and cultural processes that contribute to stigma and providing evidence-based interventions to combat it. Chapters critically investigate the ideological and instrumental barriers to mental healthcare and establish that determining the conceptualisations of mental illness helps to unravel the reasons for the underutilisation of mental health services. A compelling case is made for a complementary healthcare model and bottom-up approach that is sensitive to the spiritual and cultural needs of the people.

The text's specific examination of mental healthcare in African countries makes it a timely piece for assisting mental health professionals in understanding the inequities in care that Black, Asian and Minority Ethnic (BAME) groups face and how to improve mental healthcare and delivery to these groups.

Ugo Ikwuka, PhD, lectures at the University of Wolverhampton, UK. He has published several works on causal attributions for mental illness, pathways to mental healthcare, and barriers to accessing mental healthcare.

Living with Mental Illness in a Globalised World

Combating Stigma and Barriers to Healthcare

Ugo Ikwuka

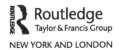

Routledge
Taylor & Francis Group

NEW YORK AND LONDON

First published 2021
by Routledge
52 Vanderbilt Avenue, New York, NY 10017

and by Routledge
2 Park Square, Milton Park, Abingdon, Oxon, OX14 4RN

Routledge is an imprint of the Taylor & Francis Group, an informa business

© 2021 Ugo Ikwuka

Library of Congress Cataloging-in-Publication Data
Names: Ikwuka, Ugo, author.
Title: Living with mental illness in a globalised world: Combating stigma and barriers to healthcare / Ugo Ikwuka.
Description: New York, NY: Routledge, 2021. | Includes bibliographical references and index. | Summary: "Living with Mental Illness in a Globalised World systematically examines the manifold contributions to the burdens of living with mental illness in a developing and globalised world. It explores the stigma of mental illness, the burden of which compares to the symptoms of and is sometimes considered more disabling than the illness itself. The book starts by reviewing the socio-psychological and cultural processes that contribute to stigma and providing evidence-based interventions to combat it. Chapters critically investigate the ideological and instrumental barriers to mental healthcare and establish that determining the conceptualisations of mental illness helps to unravel the reasons for the underutilisation of mental health services. A compelling case is made for a complementary healthcare model and bottom-up approach that is sensitive to the spiritual and cultural needs of the people. The text's specific examination of mental healthcare in African countries makes it a timely piece for assisting mental health professionals in understanding the inequities in care that Black Asian and Minority Ethnic groups face and how to improve mental healthcare and delivery to these groups"-- Provided by publisher.
Identifiers: LCCN 2020051391 (print) | LCCN 2020051392 (ebook) | ISBN 9780367698317 (hardback) | ISBN 9780367698294 (paperback) | ISBN 9781003143475 (ebook)
Subjects: LCSH: Mental illness--Social aspects. | Mentally ill--Public opinion. | Stigma (Social psychology)
Classification: LCC RC455.I42 2021 (print) | LCC RC455 (ebook) | DDC 362.19689--dc23
LC record available at https://lccn.loc.gov/2020051391
LC ebook record available at https://lccn.loc.gov/2020051392

ISBN: 978-0-367-69831-7 (hbk)
ISBN: 978-0-367-69829-4 (pbk)
ISBN: 978-1-003-14347-5 (ebk)

Typeset in Times New Roman
by MPS Limited, Dehradun

To

Esbito

Contents

Foreword   x
Preface   xiii
Acknowledgements   xvi

PART I
Attitudes towards Mental Illness   1
  Introduction 1

1 The Socio-psychological Processes of Stigma   3

2 Types of Mental Illness Stigma   8
  Public Stigma 8
  Self-stigma 10
  Associative Stigma 11

3 Stigma Predisposing Factors   14
  Culture 14
  Causal Explanations for Mental Illness 16
  (Mis)conceptualisation and (Mis)representation of
  Mental Illness 19
  Nature and Symptom Presentation of Illness 22
  Diagnosis of Mental Illness and Psychiatric
  Hospitalisation 23

4 Consequences of the Stigma of Mental Illness   25
  Social Exclusion 25
  Structural Discrimination 30
  Increased Burden of Disease 32
  Impedance of Help-seeking 33
  Impedance of Treatment and Recovery 35

5 **Pervasiveness of Stigma**   38
   The Developing World 38
   The Developed World 41
   Demographic Correlates of Stigmatising Attitudes 43

6 **Improving Stigmatising Attitudes**   48
   Education 48
   Contact 51
   Advocacy 55
   A Multi-dimensional Approach 62

PART II
Barriers to Mental Healthcare   63
   Introduction 63

7 **Help-Seeking Determinants and Ideological Barriers**   65
   The Sociocultural Context 65
   The Conceptualisation of Disease 68
   Cultural (In)appropriateness of Care 71
   Mental Health Literacy 76
   Culture of Self-reliance 79
   Stigma of Mental Illness 80

8 **Help-Seeking Determinants and Instrumental Barriers**   81
   The Social Network 81
   Experience of the Mental Health System 85
   Inadequacy of Services 91
   Case for Integrated Primary Care 95

9 **Ideological vs. Instrumental Barriers**   100
   Barriers to Help-seeking: Socio-demographic
   Correlates 100

PART III
Pathways to Mental Healthcare: Evolving an Effective
Design   107
   Introduction 107

10 **Pathways to Mental Healthcare**   109
   The Biomedical Model 109

The 'Free Market' Model 109
    Spiritual Pathway (Faith Healers) 110
    Traditional Pathway 1 111
    Traditional Pathway 2: The Social Network 111

11 **Patterns of Mental Healthcare Pathways in
    Sub-Saharan Africa**   112

12 **Conclusion: Towards a Complementary Model of Mental
    Healthcare**   117

    References   122
    Subject index   165

Foreword

The importance of mental health to overall wellbeing is now well accepted by policymakers. Mental disorders alongside other non-communicable diseases such as cancer, cardiovascular disease and diabetes cause 70% of deaths globally. Depression, probably the most common mental disorder, is currently among the ten leading causes of disability-adjusted life years (DALYs) and is projected to be among the top three by 2030 (Mathers & Loncar, 2006). Estimates of years lived with disability in 2017 confirmed that low back pain, headache disorders and depression were the top three conditions in both males and females, globally (GBD, 2017; Disease and Injury Incidence and Prevalence Collaborators, 2018). The direct human effect of these facts is exemplified by suicide figures: suicide is the leading cause of death in young people aged 15–29 years and is in the top three leading causes of death among those aged 15–44 years. In 2016, 79% of suicides occurred in low- and middle-income countries (WHO, 2020).

It is in this context that Ugo Ikwuka's book *Living with mental illness in a globalised world* makes its arrival. It is an in-depth study indeed. It is a comprehensive and thoughtful account of the burden of mental illness stigma, and the social and cultural barriers that impede access to mental health service globally, but especially in low- and middle-income countries. Even though there is a focus on Nigeria and sub-Saharan Africa, many of its lessons have pancultural generality.

Let me say, any discussion about barriers to accessing mental health services must first underline the absolute paucity of mental health services in general and emphasise its poor relation to physical health services. And, culture matters too, because it contributes to health disparities by structuring inequalities and the distribution of health problems and resources. It is usual and unsurprising to acknowledge that culture influences disease symptomatology, the course and outcome of disease, the shaping of individual and family coping mechanisms and adaptation to illness, and in determining help-seeking behaviour and finally the nature of patient-doctor relationships.

But, less well recognised is the degree to which culture frames the values that underpin healthcare decision-making. In other words, the sharp disparities on budgetary provisions for mental health services compared to physical health is a sad reflection of the position of mental disorders in the public mind and the influence of this on policymakers and politicians' decisions. This is a proper subject for study, and Ikwuka focuses our attention on what stigma is and how it adversely influences healthcare systems by determining the nature of social exclusion, structuring discrimination, increasing the burden of disease and impeding both help-seeking behaviour and recovery.

An examination of the Millennium Development Goals (MDGs) including the eradication of hunger and poverty, achieving universal primary education, promoting gender equality, reducing child mortality, improving maternal health and so on quickly demonstrates the astonishing absence of any goals relating to mental disorders, despite the ubiquity and gravity of these conditions and their impact on life expectancy and mortality. It is, of course, impossible for any human being to flourish in the absence of mental well-being. Thankfully, it is now an accepted maxim that 'there is no health without mental health.' This maxim cements the facts that mental disorders contribute considerable burdens to individuals and their families, make significant contributions to mortality and reduced life expectancy, and that there are multi-faceted inter-connections between mental illness and physical disorders.

Finally, I want to draw attention to the World Health Organisation's Project Atlas (WHO, 2018). The domains include governance, policies, plans, laws, financing and payment systems, services and resources. I want to focus attention on the immense disparities between low-, lower-middle-, and upper-middle-income countries on the one hand and high-income countries on the other. The differences are as great as 1.3 hospital beds/100,000 population to 30.9 beds/100,000, for example, in the provision of hospital beds.

These disparities are further amplified by the lack or absence of nurses, psychologists, occupational therapists and psychiatrists. Significant gaps in funding underpin these disparities: Nigeria, for example, spends $97 per head of population on healthcare per annum and only a fraction of this is spent on mental health services. The United Kingdom spends $4,192 per head of population and the United States $9,892. It is clear that whatever impediments culture contributes to the distinctly poor access to care, impoverished services make a more than significant contribution to the parlous state of affairs.

Ugo Ikwuka's book is an extraordinary achievement. It forensically interrogates the field, and it is the only book to my knowledge that systematically examines and records the manifold contributions to the burdens of living with mental disorder in a globalised world. It is sensitively written and with deep insight. I feel very privileged to be associated with it.

Prof Femi Oyebode MBBS, MD, PhD, FRCPsych, (Hon)FRCPsych
Professor of Psychiatry, University of Birmingham & Consultant
Psychiatrist, National Centre for Mental Health Birmingham Former
Chief Examiner, Royal College of Psychiatrists

Preface

"I came back from the toilet once and this bloke making a nice comment about how I looked. Then this other bloke went, 'Oh no, she's a nutter, you don't want to go there!' and I heard them say it, and I said, 'Oh, I'm a nutter am I?' I said. 'Well, how come I can have a serious conversation with you then?' I've done this, I've done that. I really pointed him up on it, what it was really like to be labelled a nutter … It's the fear of the unknown. Once you get a label" (Crawford & Brown, 2002).

"The fear of the unknown" aptly captures the vulnerability of living with mental illness both in terms of the symptoms and the stigma. The burden is worsened in the developing world where sufferers additionally face destitution and sub-standard care. It is against this background that this book systematically examines the burdens of living with mental illness in a rapidly globalised world where many suffer mental illness dislocated from their universe of meaning.

The burden of the stigma of mental illness has been compared to that of the symptoms and is considered arguably more disabling. As culture influences the experience, expression, and determinants of stigma, and the effectiveness of different approaches to stigma reduction, any meaningful intervention to combat stigma needs to take into consideration the cultural context. This book responds to this unmet need. It systematically examines stigma from a global perspective to the context of the developing world, highlighting the contributory factors and how these adversely impact the quality of life, service provision and uptake. The book provides clear and practical steps for stigma reduction.

Meanwhile, it is projected that common mental disorders will soon disable more people than complications arising from AIDS, heart disease, traffic accidents and wars combined. Such a disturbing trajectory notwithstanding, the mental health needs of people do not translate into seeking or receiving professional help. While less than 3% of GDP is spent on health and less than 1% of this is allocated to mental healthcare in some low- and low-middle income countries, more disturbing is the realisation that most people with mental health challenges receive no mental health treatment even when care is free.

Thus, this book explores the ideological and instrumental barriers to mental healthcare both from a global perspective and in the context of the developing world. More pertinently, it robustly interrogates the factors that influence health-seeking behaviour and compliance in migrant groups. This should enable health systems to ensure equity of access and equality, especially given the growing concerns about inequities in health for Black, Asian and Minority Ethnic (BAME) groups.

Research also underscores the complexity of life in developing (traditional and borderline) societies that live harmoniously with experiences that border on contradictions when viewed from the perspective of Western psychology and psychiatry. This is reflected in the mixed (biomedical, psychosocial and supernatural) causal attributions for mental illness and the mixed preference of biomedical, spiritual and traditional healing methods in these societies. Here, cultural conceptions of the mind remain interwoven with a variety of religious beliefs as well as the ecological and social world. Insistence on a linear or 'logical' (Western) approach to care in these contexts could therefore alienate sufferers. This concern is especially heightened by the globalisation of Western culture, which presents just one version of human nature – one set of ideas about pain and suffering – as being definitive.

To achieve therapeutic alliances and meet the cultural expectations of outcome in these contexts, this book makes a compelling case for a complementary healthcare model that is sensitive to the spiritual and cultural needs of the people. While the pragmatics of such an integrated model of care must be determined, training to promote improved cultural competency of local mental health professionals would be a good starting point towards a bottom-up approach that recognises the importance of local conceptualisations of mental health difficulties for optimal service delivery.

This book is well researched and evidence-driven. While it will be particularly of interest in the field of mental healthcare, it has a very strong cross-disciplinary appeal including for psychologists, sociologists, social workers, occupational therapists, medical sociologists, pastoral counsellors, and academics with interests in the humanities and anthropology. The book will be valuable for clinicians in understanding the impact of stigma on the clinical presentation of their clients, and in discerning how to deal with the problems. It will also enlighten clinicians on cultural competency and cultural appropriateness of care. It will be a valuable resource for policymakers, mental health advocates, administrators and individuals or groups who are responsible for the organisation of mental healthcare.

This book will also inform the general reading public, including those seeking a better understanding of factors that impede progress in societal understanding and support for those with mental health difficulties. It will improve the understanding of those who care for persons with mental illness and equally enlighten sufferers themselves, especially helping to mitigate self-stigma. This text will be very resourceful for undergraduate and postgraduate scholars as well as teachers and practitioners in healthcare, especially mental healthcare, as a primary or supplementary source.

Ugo Ikwuka, PhD, London

Acknowledgements

I'm grateful to mentors and professional colleagues: Niall Galbraith, Ken Manktelow, Jo Chen-Wilson, Femi Oyebode, Lovemore Nyatanga, Abiodun Adewuya, Anuli Igboaka, Rosemary Muomah and Elly Phillips. I equally appreciate the support of my families: Ikwuka, Nwawulu, Spiritans, and the goodwill of my friends: Ken, Chidi, Malachy, Austin N., Mike, Fabian, Damasus, Uche, Jude, Raymond, Arinze, Obinna, Austin O., Fidel and Oby, Emma and Mary, Steve and Ify, Emeka and Nkiru, Paul and Ijeoma, Ikenna and Esther, Bob and Aku, Vin and Rosebells, Johnny and Oby, Mike and Edith, Lawrence and Ozioma, Fidel and Ere, Ken and UK, Johnny and Odii, Jude and Beatrice, Essien and Patricia, Nsikan and Gloria, Inno and Betty, Ernest, Pat, Ikenna, Gab, Tonia, Danielle, Stella, Buife, Uche, Chinelo, Ijeoma, Joe, KC, Florian, Maria, Tim, Juliea, Ignatius, Tony, Maureen, Mary, Joan and a host of others. I am especially very grateful to Dr Petronilla Tabansi, Sally Staples and Michael Kelly for painstakingly reviewing the book drafts.

Part I

Attitudes towards Mental Illness

Introduction

Mental illness remains highly stigmatised worldwide (Morris et al., 2018). The form and nature may differ across cultures, but stigmatisation of mental illness is present in all societies and all classes of people. In almost all settings, whether social or professional, persons suffering from mental disorders will most certainly endure bigotry, ostracism, prejudice, a diminished social and economic standing, a lowered self-esteem and self-worth (Corrigan & Rao, 2012; Markowitz, 2014; Wu, Chang, Chen, Wang, & Lin, 2015). The burden of the stigma of mental illness has been compared to that of the symptoms and is considered arguably more disabling (Coker, 2005; Feldman & Crandall, 2007; Hinshaw & Stier, 2008), thus constituting double jeopardy for sufferers.

Research interest in the role of stigma in mental health has heightened as mental health-related problems have been accentuated in the public consciousness by celebrities and global leaders alike. Culture influences the experience, expression, and determinants of stigma, and the effectiveness of different approaches to stigma reduction (Al-Krenawi, Graham, Al-Bedah, Kadri, & Sehwail, 2009). Any meaningful intervention to combat stigma, therefore needs to take into consideration the cultural context. However, an unmet need for further research into the phenomenon has been noted, especially in the developing world where mental illness is suffered against the background of destitution and substandard care (Bhugra, 2006; Yang, 2007).

Rather than keeping a captive clientele in hospitals, deinstitutionalisation policies – a process that involves replacing long-stay psychiatric hospitals with less isolated community mental health services has become the major strategic response of national governments to coping with mental illness. The policy is supported by the strong evidence of 'institutionalism' – the development of disabilities as a consequence of social isolation and institutional care in remote asylums (Thornicroft & Tansella, 2002).

Consequently, the role of the community in the prevention of mental illness and care of afflicted persons has become acknowledged as the most

appropriate basis for the development of community mental health programmes (Dessoki & Hifnawy, 2009). As deinstitutionalisation equally
entails initiatives for public education on the recognition and prevention
of mental conditions and the promotion of mental health in the population (Arboleda-Flórez, 2001), the knowledge of public attitudes to mental
illness and its treatment becomes crucial to the realisation of successful
community-based programmes.

The World Psychiatric Association (2002) acknowledged that the assessment of the community attitude to mental illness, and surveys of
target groups with defined attributes are required to implement effective
educational and anti-stigma programmes. The first part of this study
robustly responds to the foregoing with a systematic account of stigma
processes, types, determinants, consequences, and prevalence. The section
concludes with evidence-based stigma reduction interventions.

1 The Socio-psychological Processes of Stigma

Attitudes are evaluative dispositions that can influence behaviour (Zimbardo & Leippe, 1991). They can help people to process complex information about the world around them. However, when formed with prejudice, attitudes can undermine that critical process of making sense of the world. For instance, they can lead to stigmatising and socially devaluing a person. Corrigan and Watson (2002) proposed a stigma concept based on stereotypes, prejudice, and discrimination. While stereotypes represent notions of groups, people who are prejudiced endorse negative stereotypes thereby generating emotional (e.g., hatred) and consequent behavioural (e.g., discrimination) reactions. Thus, attitudes always involve cognitions, emotions, and behaviours.

The ancient Greeks originally used the term stigma to represent the marks that were pricked on slaves to demonstrate ownership and to reflect their inferior social status. 'Stig' is the ancient Greek word for 'prick' and the resulting mark is 'stigma'. Thus, the stigma process consists of two fundamental components: the recognition of the differentiating 'mark' and the subsequent devaluation of the bearer. Sociological theories provide further insight into the dynamics of mental illness stigma. Erving Goffman's (1967) classic formulation relies on two constructs: the actor and the audience. The actor in this context is someone who might have a mental health problem, while the rest of the society: neighbours, employers, family members, significant others, or institutions constitute the audience. Stigma occurs when a person's actual social identity falls short of the ideal identity defined by society, such as behavioural expectations in given situations. Hence, a person with mental illness who may demonstrate lapses in social integration is a potential candidate for stigma.

Once spotted, such persons are labelled - formally tagged, which effectively isolates them. Subsequently, they are associated with undesirable characteristics, and broadly discriminated against as a result. Attitudes towards them change to agree with the label -a 'psycho' is dangerous; hence he is given a distance. Through a systematic, ongoing process of labelling and discrimination, the 'career' of mental illness is perpetuated for victims as the process effectively restricts and confines them to the world defined for them (Scheff, 1966). Discrimination in a range of spheres tacitly constrains them from returning to conventional roles. The victim is thus literally disabled: disempowered and depersonalised.

Consequently, such individuals may be compelled to interpret their experiences in the light of the prevailing social stereotype of mental illness and even modify their behaviour to fit the image. Thus, once the label is assigned, justified or not, it can become a self-fulfilling prophecy that promotes the development of psychiatric symptoms. Below, a survivor of schizophrenia relays this experience:

> Like any worthwhile endeavour, becoming a schizophrenic requires a long period of rigorous training. My training for this unique calling began in earnest when I was six years old. At that time, my somewhat befuddled mother took me to the University of Washington to be examined by psychiatrists in order to find out what was wrong with me. These psychiatrists told my mother: "We don't know exactly what is wrong with your son, but whatever it is, it is very serious. We recommend that you have him committed immediately or else he will be completely psychotic within less than a year." My mother did not have me committed since she realised that such a course of action will be extremely damaging to me. But after that ominous prophecy my parents began to view and treat me as if I were either insane or at least in the process of becoming that way. Once, when my mother caught me playing with some vile muck I had mixed up – I was seven at the time – she gravely told me, "They have people put away in mental institutions for doing things like that." Fear was written all over my mother's face as she told me this.... The slightest odd behaviour on my part was enough to send my parents into paroxysms of apprehension. My parents' apprehension in turn made me fear I was going insane.... My fate had been sealed not by my genes, but by the attitudes, beliefs, and expectations of my parents.... I find it extremely difficult to condemn my parents for behaving as if I were going insane when the psychiatric authorities told them that this was an absolute certainty.
>
> (Modrow, 2003, pp. 1–3).

Thus, the judgments of others can turn innocuous miscues into pathological symptoms, thereby reinforcing the belief that some factors of mental illness could be socially constructed. Scheff (1966) was convinced that traditional approaches to understanding mental health and illness have a narrow and incomplete focus. He contests the reductionist approach with genetic and biochemical investigations that focus somewhat exclusively on dynamic systems within the individual, while social processes and the social system in which the individual is involved tend to be undermined or at best relegated to a subsidiary role.

As demonstrated in the classic Rosenhan (1973) study, a person labelled 'mentally ill' is likely to be stigmatised even in the absence of any aberrant behaviour. In the study, eight people without mental health problems presented themselves at various psychiatric hospitals, complaining that they had been hearing voices utter the words 'empty', 'hollow', and 'thud'. They were quickly diagnosed as suffering from schizophrenia, and all eight were hospitalised. Although the false patients later dropped all their symptoms and behaved normally, they had great difficulty getting rid of the label and gaining release from the hospital. They reported that staff members were authoritarian in their behaviour towards patients, spent limited time interacting with them, and responded curtly and uncaringly to questions. In fact, they generally treated patients as though they were non-persons and invisible. One of the 'patients' recalls that a nurse unbuttoned her uniform to adjust her brassiere in the presence of an entire ward of viewing men. There was not the sense that she was being seductive (as cited in Comer, 2015).

In a study of the attitude of medical students in a south-western Nigerian University towards psychiatric label (Ogunsemi, Odusan, & Olatawura, 2008), a case vignette was presented that ended with a psychiatric label for the experimental group while the control group had the same vignette without the label. The case vignette reads, "Mr AB is a young man who can express his feelings and thoughts among those close to him, although he sometimes gets anxious while talking in a group consisting of strangers. He gets along all right with his family most of the time. Generally, he also gets along with other people. Compared to those of his age, his life can be considered as organised. He is generally an optimistic and happy person. In summary, he establishes a good balance between his social life and study". For the students in the experimental group, the vignette concluded with the additional label, "This young man has been diagnosed as having mental illness by the doctor who examined him."

Compared to those in the control group without the attached label, the students in the experimental group, who responded to the questionnaire with the attached psychiatric label, were significantly more unwilling to rent out their houses to the man. They were significantly more unwilling to have him as their next-door neighbour, barber, or hairdresser compared with the control group. They were also not willing to share an office with him or allow their sister to get married to him. They significantly felt that the man would exhaust them both physically and emotionally in their relationship with him compared to those in the control group.

Labelling defines patients in terms of their illness: 'mental patients', 'the mentally ill', 'psychotic vagrant' – terms that evoke images of chronic psychopathology. It strips sufferers of their pre-morbid identity and imposes on them the new stigmatised identity and role which comes to define them over and beyond their other roles such as parent or professional. A study of terms used by school children in England for mental illness revealed 250 different words and phrases, none of which are positive (Rose, Thornicroft, Pinfold, & Kassam, 2007). Similarly, a study that investigated school children's perception of people with mental illness in south-western Nigeria found the most popular descriptor to be derogatory terms (33%), followed by 'abnormal appearance and behaviour' (29.6%) (Ronzoni, Dogra, Omigbodun, Bella, & Atitola, 2010).

As individuals so labelled come to accept the label, they can be 'rewarded' for affirming the label by misbehaving to expectation, a process that inadvertently works to reinforce and perpetuate the 'career' of mental illness. A classic illustration is the case of Mr Spell. This ostensibly mentally challenged Nigerian spews out letters randomly to 'spell' any word. As he does this, the amused audience urges him on after each syllable, and he randomly churns out scores of letters to 'spell' a mere four-letter word. As he is excitedly urged on, he feels that he is making sense and the more he 'performs'. Moreover, his disability means that he lives on the handouts from his audience to whom he is indebted for his survival, and their support largely depends on the extent that he 'entertains' them. In fact, if for any reason he fails to misbehave, or his misbehaviour falls short of people's expectations, he could be punished, not only by being denied the token handouts on which he survives as a destitute vagrant but through direct harassment and victimisation. Today, Mr Spell's spelling folly has been adapted into music for entertainment, and many of his spelling clips trend on social media.

Indeed, the saying that "every village needs an idiot and every circus a clown" may well pass for Nigerian where it is common for people to create circuses and oblige the 'madman' (vagrant sufferer of psychosis) to amuse them with his regressive behaviour. In a case study of south-eastern Nigeria (Ikwuka, 2016), 77% of respondents agreed that people make fun of people with mental illness. As depicted in the Nigerian movie *Village Destroyers*, a common spectacle is crowding around the 'madman' who is obliged to fulfil expectations by dancing weirdly to the mockery tune sung for him. If he dances to expectation, he is 'rewarded', for instance, with something to eat, including degraded food. Otherwise, he could be denied such token handouts on which he lives. He could be additionally punished: flogged, kicked about or drenched in wastewater. The situation is reminiscent of the asylum era in Europe when watching people with mental illness became a popular form of amusement, and some asylums even had specially built patient-viewing galleries for the public.

Skinner and colleagues (1995) discern a hierarchy of stigma whereby inferior social statuses like 'prostitute' and 'alcoholic' are ranked with mental illness at the bottom of the hierarchy. The stigma of mental illness has been referred to as the 'ultimate stigma' (Falk, 2001), exceeding those of other conditions and stigmatised groups, including foreigners, immigrants, and those with physical disabilities, because the public perceives it as the most disabling (Economou, Gramandani, Richardson, & Stefanis, 2005; Thompson, Stuart, Bland et al., 2002).

By process of association and class identity, all mental health patients are stigmatised (Arboleda-Flórez, 2001). The individual patients, regardless of the level of impairment or disability, are lumped together into a class. Belonging to this class reinforces the stigma against the individual, as the stigmatised person is viewed stereotypically as a model of a social group rather than an individual. However, of the specific disorders that have been investigated, people with psychotic disorders or substance misuse have been the most stigmatised (Rao, Mahadevappa, Pillay et al., 2009; Griffiths, Nakane, Christensen et al., 2006) and their care most underfunded (Braff, 1992). Those with schizophrenia are more likely to additionally experience physical and verbal attacks (Dinos, Stevens, Serfaty, Weich, & King, 2004). Schizophrenia (madness in lay terms) is the modern-day equivalent of leprosy as there is no other disease that confers such social ostracism on the people afflicted and on their families (Torrey, 1995).

2 Types of Mental Illness Stigma

Public Stigma

Stigma operates at the personal, family and societal levels. Public stigma occurs when people endorse negative stereotypes and consequently discriminate against those labelled 'mentally ill' (Corrigan, Druss, & Perlick, 2014). It is mostly informed by the stereotypes of people with mental illness as dangerous and unpredictable. In the eyes of the general public, 'madness' equates to violence (Ewhrudjakpor, 2009; Hansson, Jorrnfeldt, Svedberg, & Svensson, 2013). Many hold stereotypical views of persons with mental illness in which psychotic behaviour is expected (Rogers & Pilgrim, 2010).

With the stereotype of dangerousness and unpredictability, fear becomes the primary impulse for the development of stigma (Arboleda-Flórez, 2001; American Psychological Association, 2018). This corroborates Foucault's (1978) observation that the strongest cultural stereotype of persons with mental illness focuses on the spectre of a homicidal madman – a deranged being who explodes violently, erratically and inexplicably. A real or imagined fear of aggression can therefore lead to avoidance of people with mental illness. Following the Hungerford massacre of 1987 in England, a statistically significant increase in public support for the statement 'people who commit horrific crimes, such as the murder of children or old people, are likely to be mentally ill' was reported (Appleby & Wessely, 1988).

As a rule, and for all disorders, the level of social distance desired from people with mental illness increases with the degree of 'intimacy' implied by the relationship (Gaebel, Baumann, Witte, & Zaeske, 2002; Stuart & Arboleda-Flórez, 2001a). This is corroborated in the aforementioned case study of south-eastern Nigeria (Ikwuka, 2016) whereby social distance desired at the primary (more intimate) level of association, for example in marriage, was more significantly endorsed (85.7%) compared to that desired at the secondary (less intimate) level of association, for example sharing of the neighbourhood (52.5%).

Among the Igbo people of south-eastern Nigeria, many stereotypical depictions of the 'madman' *onyeara* are couched in pejorative or, at best, patronising anecdotes of his sayings and activities. For instance, to underscore his insanity, *onyeara* is quoted to have said, "*O nweghị ihe m ga-agwa onye ji nnukwu nmà aga m n'azụ, na-abụghi mgbe m chọrọ isi m achọ*" (It is until my head goes missing that I would have something to say to the man who is carelessly brandishing a machete behind me). Another saying ascribed to the madman indicates that he has no sense of cause and effect. He was said to have ignited a fire that razed an entire estate, but when he was confronted, he explains: "*Sọ ebe m munyere ọkụ ka m ga-akọwa, ihe mere ebe ndị ọzọ agbasaghị m ma ncha*" (I can only account for the spot where I struck the match, whatever happened beyond that has nothing to do with me).

Yet, another stereotype presents *onyeara* as lacking a sense of proportionate action. He was said to have knocked on someone's door but to have got no response, presumably because the occupants saw him as a nuisance. When time went on, and the door was not answered, he set the house on fire (to attract the attention of the occupants) and then declared: "*Ndị nwe ụlọ na-anọghi ya, mgbe nta ha ga-anọ ya*" (The occupants of the house who are supposedly unavailable will soon emerge inexplicably).

Illustrating the idea that persons with mental illness lack self-control and are unpredictable, *onyeara* was said to have declared: "*Ihe kpatara eji akpọ m onyeara bụ maka na m chọọ ikwu ọzọ, ọzọ apụta m n'ọnụ*" (Why they call me mad is because, when I want to say one thing, another pops out of my mouth). A patronising stereotype of persons with mental illness which people in the region use to describe the uncertainties in their own lives is expressed in the proverb where the madman is said to have declared: "*Ihe kpatara m ji agba-ụzọ abughi maka na ebe m na-aga di anya, kama, ọ bụ adi ama ama, tinyere igba egwu mberede nwere ike idapụtara m n'ọma ahia*" (I hasten, not because my target destination is far away, but because of the possibility of unforeseen circumstances, including the probability of my stopping to dance at the market square).

Another anecdote that patronises the 'wisdom' of the madman holds that as he was passing by a church, he overheard the preacher announce that he would be reading St. Paul's Letter to the Corinthians (a book in the Bible). He quickly dashed into the church to openly question the morality of reading someone's letter to the public. He then threatened that, as a punishment for the people's misdemeanour, he was going to set many houses in the community ablaze. This brought the church service to an abrupt end as people scurried home to protect their houses.

Such stereotypical depictions of persons with mental illness could also suggest that they are incapable of normal human lines of thought. Aside the stereotype of dangerousness endorsed by 88% of the respondents, a study by the Canadian Mental Health Association (1994) found the most prevalent misconceptions about persons with mental illness to include that they had a low IQ or were developmentally handicapped (40%), could not function, hold down a job, or had anything to contribute (32%)

and lacked will power or were weak or lazy (24%). This is echoed in a related study (Stuart & Arboleda-Flórez, 2001b) where 72% of the respondents believed that persons with schizophrenia could not work in regular jobs.

Arboleda-Flórez (2001) cites Michelle, a vivacious 25-year-old office worker, who shared her major disappointment with her family and family friends who simply expected her to have an abortion when she announced that she was pregnant. They assumed that her schizophrenia would incapacitate her to deliver and to care for her baby. They were also afraid that her medications could have teratogenic effects on the baby. She carried her baby to term and took care of it despite the opposition of family and friends.

Self-stigma

Self-stigma is a transformation process whereby one's previously held identity is supplanted by a stigmatised less desirable view of one's self. The shift from public to self-stigma occurs when negative associations determine an individual's sense of their own self rather than the opinion of a group (Austin & Goodman, 2017). Thus, persons with mental illness stigmatise themselves when they internalise or embody the corresponding prejudice, and succumbing to the negative profile imposed on them, they become prejudiced towards themselves. Internalised stigma is related to feelings of mortification and humiliation for having a mental disorder (Wu, Chang, Chen, Wang, & Lin, 2015). It can lead to low self-esteem (Marcussen, Gallagher, & Ritter, 2018; Ritsher & Phelan, 2004), self-loathing (Larson & Corrigan, 2008), avoidance of social activities (Perlick et al., 2001), depression (Leff & Warner, 2006), a sense of shame, fear and loneliness (Granerud & Severinsson, 2006). Ultimately, these result in a low quality of life. Patients may become captives in their homes because of neighbours' twitching curtains, whispering about them and cold-shouldering. It could also lead to concealment of psychiatric conditions, living in denial of symptoms, and fear and discouragement from promptly seeking appropriate treatment.

Those who live in denial of their symptoms or concealment of their conditions may be considerably stressed in managing the disguise. Furthermore, because some mental health difficulties are often not obvious to the casual observer, the sufferer may be very wary of anything that might give them away and is thus in perpetual conflict. Yet, if their condition inadvertently manifests, for instance, in episodes of crisis, they subsequently face the arduous task of perpetually 'mending face' (Goffman, 1967). Living with such an unsettled internal state, they are less likely to be successful at work and in relationships. It could lead to defensive and situational causal attribution for the condition by the sufferer and their family. For instance, in societies that advance supernatural causal explanations, they could allege that the condition is the handiwork of spiritual forces, or evildoers, (Aghukwa, 2009a). This could lead to rejection or discontinuation of biomedical care.

Exaggerated pessimistic attitudes about prognosis may also increase self-stigmatisation, which could lead to the evasion of help-seeking. Thus, self-stigma is a major obstacle to the recovery of those with mental illness. It compounds the effects of stigmatisation. It is considered the most damaging aspect of stigma, as the internalisation of the stigmatised status can lead mental health service users to believe that they are of less value and incapable of working and independent living (Corrigan & Penn, 1999; Green, Hayes, Dickinson, Whitaker, & Gilheaney, 2003).

One in four psychiatric patients in Nigeria has experienced high self-stigma (Adewuya, Owoeye, Erinfolami, & Ola, 2011). In *The Last Taboo* (Simmie & Nunes, 2001), one of the authors describes his feelings after a bout of major depression: "Stigma was, for me, the most agonising aspect of my disorder. It cost friendships, career opportunities, and – most importantly – my self-esteem. It wasn't long before I began internalising the attitudes of others, viewing myself as a lesser person. Many of those long days in bed during the depression were spent thinking, 'I'm mentally ill. I'm a manic-depressive. I'm not the same anymore'. I wondered desperately if I would ever work again, ever be 'normal' again. It was a god-awful feeling that contributed immensely to the suicidal yearnings that invaded my thoughts."

Associative Stigma

The impact of stigma is not limited to the person with mental illness. It can also affect their family, friends and associates through "courtesy stigma" (Corrigan & Miller, 2004). Families report lowered self-esteem and strained relationships with other family members because of stigma (Gray, 2001; van der Sanden, Bos, Stutterheim, Pryor, & Kok, 2013). Half of the families surveyed by Phelan and colleagues (1998) in the Suffolk County of New York had concealed their relative's hospitalisation from others because of the fear of social rejection.

Associative stigma is more widely felt in communitarian cultures because the family represents the centre of the social institution with the burden of the stigma resting more with the family than on the individual (Adler, & Mukheji, 1995). While emotions such as pride and shame relate to how personal behaviour reflects on the self in individualistic cultures, they relate mainly to how personal behaviour reflects on others in collectivist cultures (Mesquita, 2001). Collectivist aspects of some Asian groups, may, for example, lead to perceptions that disabilities of mental illness reflect the flaws of the family (Lauber & Rössler, 2007; Sanchez & Gaw, 2007).

Over 50% of respondents, in a study of the attitudes of 160 Yemeni men, justified their reasons for not having a relationship with someone with a mental disability on the grounds of fear that they would be viewed negatively by their peers (Alzubaidi, Baluch & Moafi, 1995). Shame is worsened when disabilities suggest lack of conformity to social norms (Lam, Tsang, Chan, & Corrigan, 2006). As a result, groups that endorse stigma are less likely to seek services when in need (Miville & Constantine, 2007; Shea & Yeh, 2008).

An Igbo adage aptly reflects associative stigma, *Nwanne onye na-agba ajọ egwu, ọkọ iku a na-akọ ya* (When someone is dancing weirdly - misbehaving, his kinsmen will suddenly develop itchy eyebrows). The scratching of 'itchy eyebrows' is metaphorical of covering their faces in shame. In the case study of south-eastern Nigeria (Ikwuka, 2016), 57.7% of respondents acknowledged that they would feel ashamed should a member of their family suffer mental illness. If a history of mental illness is found in either a potential marriage partner or one of their family members in Nigeria, the marriage would generally not proceed.

A man, whose wife suffers from schizophrenia, recalls how mental illness still attracts shame to many families in Nigeria: "My wife's mental illness started after the birth of our fourth child ... At first, I thought it was high fever but it degenerated to the point of her making trouble with everybody in the neighbourhood and going nude at times. It has been hard for us, especially me, the husband, because of the costs, work and shame that I have to bear" (Eaton & Tilly-Gyado, 2009, as cited in Ewhrudjakpor, 2010b, p. 139). Family members experiencing associative stigma often feel alienated from neighbours and co-workers (Magliano, Fiorillo, de Rosa, Malangone, & Maj, 2005; Perlick et al., 2007), the very people in a putative support network that might assist the family in its goals.

To protect the integrity of their kinship system and group identity, communitarian cultures may be led to distance themselves from the person with mental illness. Goffman (1967) had argued that the face is a sacred thing hence everyday life's ritual actions centre on protecting it. Therefore, in the light of the prevalent negative view of mental illness, the illness burden for persons with mental illness, and their relatives by association, will include the exerting psychological task of preserving or protecting 'face'. This could involve trying to conceal a relative's status or hospitalisation.

Yet, associative stigma can also be observed in the more individualistic (Western) cultures. Reporting from Canada, Arboleda-Flórez (2001) tells the story of John, a 19-year-old university student, who had to accept the termination of a relationship he had just started with a girl from his neighbourhood. Her parents objected to the relationship and decided to send her to another city for her education partly in an attempt to break up the relationship once they knew that John's mother's frequent hospitalisations for the past several years were not due to "diabetes" but to a manic-depressive illness. John described the experience with some resignation: "It seems as if I have to carry the sins of my parents." Some family members and friends can also experience vicarious stigma – the sense of sadness and helplessness a family member feels when observing a relative being the object of prejudice or discrimination because of mental illness (Corrigan & Miller, 2004).

By association, mental health practices and practitioners can also be stigmatised. A comprehensive review of more than 500 studies showed that the public endorses various stereotypes about psychiatry and psychiatrists (Sartorius et al., 2010). Psychiatrists were perceived to represent "the end of the line" and were associated with "mad people" or "asylums" (Youssef & Deane, 2006). There is an anecdotal belief that psychiatrists tend to behave like their clients. In a study, medical students reportedly believed that psychiatrists "must be crazy". They viewed psychiatric practice as having low status, the public viewed it as ineffective or possibly harmful, patients viewed it as failing to target essential problems, and the media viewed it as a discipline without true scholarship (Corrigan et al., 2014).

Psychiatrists are often stereotypically portrayed in the media as libidinous lechers, eccentric buffoons, vindictive, repressive agents of society, or evil-minded, and in the case of female psychiatrists, as loveless and unfulfilled women (Gabbard & Gabbard, 1992). Psychiatrists and psychologists are not as highly respected or appreciated and do not have the same elevated status as other medical practitioners because they work with 'mad people' (Wellington, 1992). The theory of cognitive dissonance (Festinger, 1957) suggests that, given a choice, healthcare professionals will tend to select careers in areas which attract favourable attitudes. Student psychiatric nurses reported disappointment from their family members on their choice of specialisation (Wells, McElwee, & Ryan, 2000).

A study of students in their final year of medical school in northwestern Nigeria showed that less than 2% considered psychiatry as a first choice professional pathway, more than 50% expressed social distance towards psychiatric patients, and decried poor remunerations associated with the profession (Aghukwa, 2010). A teacher in Maiduguri, northeastern Nigeria, vowed that she would never allow any of her offspring to specialise in psychiatry nor marry a psychiatrist because of the age-old cultural belief among the Kanuri people that anyone treating persons with mental illness would likely have one of their offspring suffer from a mental ailment (Oyegbile, 2009).

3 Stigma Predisposing Factors

Culture

The prevailing beliefs which shape people's notions of mental illness include stereotypes as well as the climate in which these stereotypes are endorsed (Corrigan, Druss, & Perlick, 2014). Culture provides a repertoire of affective and behavioural responses to the human condition. It influences the construction of what is normal and abnormal behaviour and the interpretation of an event as stressful (Nwokocha, 2010; Okafor, 2009; Thomas, 2008). It also offers models of how people should or might feel and act in response to the serious mental illness of a loved one (Jenkins & Karno, 1992). Dohrenwend (1966) noted that ethnically based cultural norms could shape perceptions of the social undesirability of psychiatric symptoms. They determine social indicators of mental illness, thereby impacting stigmatising cues (Abdullah & Brown, 2011). The stigma attached to psychiatric services may also be influenced by traditional health belief systems (Gellis, Huh, Lee, & Kim, 2003). As people tend to hold strong beliefs about mental illness (Asuni, Schoenberg, & Swift, 1994), if cultural beliefs surrounding psychiatry are negative, the attitudes of people towards sufferers will remain largely negative.

In individualistic cultures, behaviour is often determined by personal goals, while, in collectivist cultures, in-group goals are given greater salience. This results in the possibility of a stronger spread of negative attitudes, with families more likely to elect to keep secret the existence of a member with a disability or mental illness (Triandis, 1989). It corroborates the view that gregariousness fosters gossip and provincial attitudes of interference with personal problems in a closed and centralised system (Levav et al., 2004; Papadopoulos, Leavey, & Vincent, 2002).

Studying suicides in the Indian context, Gehlot and Nathawat (1983) found that a large number of cases could be explained by 'performance' failures which refer to the fact that when individuals fail to 'perform' or live up to expectations imposed by family and society as a whole, they experience shame, worry about social stigma with fears of having let the family/community down. As Pearce (1989) observed, aspects of group life can become noxious for an individual who finds a situation stressful as a result of them. Negative perceptions of and attitudes towards people with mental illness in Nigeria is partly linked to deeply rooted negative cultural beliefs that see mental illness as a deviation from normality (Ewhrudjakpor, 2009; Kabir, Iliyasu, Abubakar, & Aliyu, 2004).

The fundamental characteristic of stigma is 'difference' (Link & Phelan, 2001) which could be particularly pronounced with a person with mental illness who may ostensibly deviate from the norm or demonstrate lapses in social integration. 'Difference' can easily be spotted in collectivist cultures like that of the Igbo of south-eastern Nigeria, where four in five of people endorsed authoritarian attitude towards people with mental illness (Ikwuka, 2016). This attitude sees a clear difference between people with mental illness and others and proposes their immediate hospitalisation.

Deviance (difference) associated with serious mental disorders is a key trigger for negative attitudes in the conformist collectivist society. Almost all of the respondents (94.7%) in the aforementioned case study (Ikwuka, 2016) saw people with mental illness as 'different' while a similarly significant proportion (91.5%) endorsed the immediate hospitalisation of anyone who shows signs of mental illness. Levey and Howells (1995) found that people with psychotic conditions such as schizophrenia are thought of as being essentially 'different' in terms of their perceived unpredictability and dangerousness. This attitude underpins the widespread fear of schizophrenia held by many.

A great deal of stigmatisation is also attached to mental illness in cultures that emphasise saving face and bringing honour to the family (Leong & Lau, 2001). In traditionalist communitarian cultures, an individual's behaviour is perceived to be a reflection of the extent to which the whole family upholds social values, norms, and expectations (Erickson & al-Timimi, 2001). Social reputation is, therefore, a crucial factor that must not be compromised by any shameful threats. The culture of shame and saving face can thus lead to custodial care and tucking away of persons with mental illness, and, in the process, disenfranchising them of social privileges and also compromising their human rights.

Hence, while the social networks in these societies demonstrate a strong disposition towards providing support for family members when needed, they are also very intolerant of deviant behaviours. Thus, families can act as a protective shield against stress but can also be a major source of stress with their expectations of conformity. Such pervasive negative attitudes are a contradiction in the traditionally communitarian societies and are especially disturbing given the significance of the traditional solidarity shown the vulnerable in these cultures in compensating for the poor healthcare system.

Causal Explanations for Mental Illness

Explanatory Models (EMs) are the complex, culturally determined process of making sense of one's illness, ascribing meanings to symptoms, evolving causal attributions, and expressing suitable treatment expectations and related outcomes (Kleinman, 1978). Beliefs people hold about mental illness are influenced by ethnicity (Hall & Tucker, 1985), culture (Furnham & Chan, 2004; Jang, Kim, Hansen, & Chiriboga, 2007), religion (Pfeifer, 1994), and socioeconomic status (Dessoki & Hifnawy, 2009). Thus, people identify causal factors of illness that reflect the specific circumstances of their own lives.

A meta-analysis found relationships between illness perceptions and psychological distress, perceived illness consequences, low control, pessimistic prognosis, and longer timeline perceptions (Hagger & Orbell, 2003). Illness perceptions are also associated with future negative outcomes including: lack of adherence to treatment (Halm, Mora, & Leventhal, 2006; Weinman, Petrie, Sharpe, & Walker, 2000), slow recovery (Galli, Ettlin, Palla, Ehlert, & Gaab, 2010; Kaptein et al., 2010) and even mortality (Chilcot, Wellsted, & Farrington, 2011). Stigmatising attitudes towards persons with mental illness have been directly associated with explanatory models of illness causation (Gureje, Olley, Ephraim-Oluwanuga, & Kola, 2006). Poor causal knowledge is also among the defining factors that inform social distancing from patients of serious mental illness (Grausgruber, Meise, Katschnig, *Schöny*, & Fleischhacker, 2007).

Attribution theories underscore the importance of the causal beliefs people hold for a characteristic or behaviour in determining their responses to the person displaying the characteristic or behaviour (Bag, Yilmaz, & Kirpinar, 2006; Jorm & Griffiths, 2008). Generally, negative attitudes are displayed towards patients whose illnesses are believed to be caused supernaturally (Mulatu, 1999). Supernatural causal attribution, such as ancestral curses, breaking of taboo and witchcraft, that associates mental illness with forces beyond the individual, can elicit perceptions of strangeness, unpredictability and dangerousness. It could lead to the indictment of the individual who may be seen as suffering a divine punishment. It has also been associated with the persistent dehumanising use of physical restraints on people with mental illness and their isolation by society (Minas & Diatri, 2008).

A study that assessed explanatory models and health beliefs of mental illness patients in sub-Saharan Africa found that among respondents with a high perception of self-stigma, supernatural attribution predominated (70%) (Makanjuola et al., 2016). Most sub-Saharan African cultures subscribe to the belief that the root cause of psychosis is supernatural (Atilola, 2015; Abbo, Okello, Ekblad, Waako, & Musisi, 2008). The case study of south-eastern Nigeria (Ikwuka, 2016) revealed that 80.2% of respondents endorsed effects of spiritual curses (from God, ancestors, holy men/women, elders) as possible causes of mental illness, 80% endorsed committing abomination, 83.4% endorsed breaking of an oath or swearing falsely, 81% believed that mental illness could be caused by the mishandling of spiritual powers, 78.3% endorsed spiritual attacks, 81.7% endorsed occultism, 82.5% spirit possession and 35.1% bad luck.

High endorsement of supernatural causation can undermine biomedical causal explanations and engender deep-seated negative attitudes towards mental illness (Grausgruber et al., 2007; Putman, 2008; Ukpong & Abasiubong, 2010). It can also have implications for compliance with, and enforcement of the biomedical model of intervention. In the study by Makanjuola and colleagues (2016), a 37-year-old Nigerian male sufferer was convinced that seeking care from biomedical sources was a waste of time, based on his conviction that his mental illness was of supernatural origin: "It was so strange to me, and this makes me to believe that there is spiritual attack, and most of these madness (mad people) that roamed the street are not responsible for their plight but have been afflicted by spiritual attack, and this is the reason it is difficult to cure because it cannot be medically cured, it cannot be cured with medical ways of treatment but in traditional ways."

While there was a clear trend with the biopsychosocial explanatory models of illness being more commonly employed by low scorers on the stigma scale in the sub-Saharan Africa study (Makanjuola et al., 2016), there were respondents with a high perception of self-stigma who advanced biopsychosocial reasons for their illness. For instance, a 40-year-old male respondent from Kenya considered that the illness could be a consequence of stress resulting from coping mechanisms being overwhelmed: "What I think is that too much stress and thoughts could have caused the mental illness too. You know your thoughts are determined by the amount of problems you have – you can be having a problem that you can't even solve and it eats you up." Similarly, a 33-year-old Nigerian male respondent with a high perception of self-stigma reported anxiety about a job promotion being the cause of his illness: "Well, what caused it was that I was very young then, my former job required more experience than I possessed then for me to be promoted ... so the anxiety for promotion caused my sickness."

Studies of German and Russian samples (Dietrich et al., 2004) also indicate that endorsing biological factors as the cause of schizophrenia is associated with a greater desire for social distance. Considering the condition as coming from a stable trait can lead to pessimism about prognosis and treatment outcome. There can equally be a concern that through defective genes, the condition could be subsequently inflicted on offspring (Read, 2007), thus exacerbating the dimensions of associative stigma experienced by relatives. The case study of south-eastern Nigeria (Ikwuka, 2016) observed that a significant proportion of respondents made biogenetic causal attribution for mental illness, with 84.9% endorsing heredity. This perhaps explains why as much as 81.8% of the same sample indicated that they would not marry someone who had been cured of mental illness. Biogenetic attributions can also fuel the stereotype of un-predictability since, located in one's genes, the condition could be considered to be beyond the sufferer's control.

Moreover, attributing their condition to a biochemical aberration renders persons with mental illness as different – a determinant factor in the stigma process (see Culture above). Such evidence-based causal factors as biogenetics should therefore be advanced cautiously, recognising their potential implication for stigma. Indeed, aetiologically, there has been some controversy in the literature surrounding whether changing attitudes towards or away from a medical model is desirable in decreasing stigma (Pitre, Stewart, Adams, Bedard, & Landry, 2007). A meta-analysis of 33 reports on 16 population studies from around the world showed a steady increase in the perception of mental illness as a treatable biological disorder, yet the stigma of depression remained constant during this time while that of schizophrenia significantly worsened (Schomerus et al., 2012).

The increasing endorsement of the use of illicit drugs and alcohol as causal factors for mental illness in sub-Saharan Africa, when linked to the moral failings on the part of the users, is associated with a stigmatising and negative attitude towards people with mental illness (Crabb et al., 2012). Reinforced by the strong belief of many African cultures in retributive justice, when mental illness is associated with the recklessness of substance misuse, the sufferers can be seen as paying for their sins. Such a belief deprives them of the sympathy and understanding traditionally bestowed on the sick in the communitarian African society.

Research further reveals the interaction of culture and causal explanations in shaping attitudes towards people with mental illness. For instance, in India, reduced social distance for both depression and psychosis was consistently associated with the belief that the problems are caused by personal weakness (Kermode, Bowen, Arole, Pathare, & Jorm, 2009). In contrast, positive association between social distance and viewing mental disorders as a sign of personal weakness is found in surveys of a number of Western samples including: Australia (Jorm & Griffiths, 2008), USA (Martin, Pescosolido, Olafsdottir, & McLeod, 2007), the Netherlands (van't Veer, Kraan, Drosseart, & Modde, 2006) and Austria (Grausgruber et al., 2007).

While the majority of studies of Western samples (Jorm & Oh, 2009) indicated a negative association between psychodynamic causal explanations (childhood adversity/social stressors) and social distance, a study of a Turkish population (Ozmen et al., 2004) found a positive association. Furthermore, while all the studies of Western populations in the review by Jorm and Oh (2009) found a positive association between biogenetic causal explanations and social distance, the USA (Martin et al., 2007) and the Netherlands (van't Veer et al., 2006) were two exceptions.

Interestingly too, there were respondents in the Makanjuola and colleagues' (2016) study who made a high endorsement of supernatural causations but who had a low perception of self-stigma. However, these revealed a consistent theme of the illness being a sort of religious experience, with the positive narrative of their being called to serve God or some manifestation of being supernaturally gifted. Moreover, a 30-year-old-male Ghanaian respondent in the study reported both biopsychosocial and supernatural causes: "Sometimes it is caused by alcohol, cannabis, stealing and sometimes people can buy it for you (i.e. one can be afflicted or attacked spiritually)."

Thus, given the complexity of the interaction between explanatory models of causation and perceptions of stigma, clear-cut interventions designed to reduce or minimise stigma may, of themselves, be insufficient. Makanjuola and colleagues also rightly noted that despite previous associations of supernatural explanatory models with poorer insight and more psychopathology, and the obvious desirability of the biopsychosocial model by western trained psychiatrists, interventions designed to educate against supernatural explanatory models need to be embraced with caution. This is especially as the base or support upon which the self-esteem of some patients stand may be inadvertently eroded, leading to despondency, hopelessness, and suicide.

(Mis)conceptualisation and (Mis)representation of Mental Illness

Psychosis is, by far, the most easily recognisable form of mental disorder by the lay public (Sorsdahl et al., 2009). The conceptualisation of mental illness mainly in terms of severe psychotic disorders in most of sub-Saharan Africa (Atilola & Olayiwola, 2011; Igbinomwanhia, James, & Omoaregba, 2013) is a potential basis for strong stigmatisation of mental disorders. Similarly fuelling strong negative attitudes in the region is the pervasive pessimism of prognosis that sees mental illness as incurable (Aghukwa 2009b; Botha, Koen, & Niechaus, 2006; Paterson, 2006) and terminal (Ewhrudjakpor, 2009). Studies demonstrate that increased treatability and recovery is strongly associated with positive attitudes towards mental illness (Naeem, Ayub, & Javid, 2006).

The media, which tends to be more concerned with audience sentiments and ratings rather than the social responsibility of responsible framing, is characteristically awash with exaggerated stereotypes of persons with mental illness that reinforce causal myths, prejudices, misconceptions, fear, and anxieties. The most common causes of mental illness as depicted in Nigerian (Nollywood) movies are supernatural or preternatural forces (sorcery and enchantment by witches and wizards) and repercussions of evil deeds, with effective treatment portrayed as arising mostly through spiritual means or traditional forms of care (Aroyewun-Adekomaiya & Aroyewun, 2019;

Atilola & Olayiwola, 2011). This is an industry considered the second largest in the world (UNESCO Institute for Statistics, 2009) which makes the potential impact of such (mis)representation very significant.

The grotesque and sensationalistic portrayal of persons with mental illness in the media and the movies around the world has persisted right from the beginning of the industry in the early 1900s (Francis, Pirkis, Dunt, & Blood, 2001). Wahl and Harman (1989) found that 85.6% of relatives of persons with mental illness identified movies about "mentally ill killers" as the most important contributor to the stigma of the illness. Common media depictions of persons with mental illness include: being dangerous to others, involved with crime, vulnerable and unpredictable. Such depictions stem from the sensational reporting of crimes purportedly committed by someone with a mental illness, or from movies in which a popular plot, long exploited by the cinematographic industry, is that of the "psycho killer" (Byrne, 1998).

Characters with mental illness are portrayed in prime-time TV shows as rebellious homicidal maniacs with childlike perceptions of the world. They are projected as free spirits that lack social identity, usually single, unemployed and described negatively with adjectives such as "aggressive" "confused" and "unpredictable" (Farina, 1998; Wahl, 1995). Media misrepresentations of mental illness, including in children's cartoons, and in the language employed to deplore misbehaving politicians or public officials can cause, fuel, and perpetuate both public and self-stigma. Since much of the public image of severe mental illness is informed by the mass media (Torrey, 1994; Wahl, 1995), the type of information provided by the media will be crucial in forming attitudes.

Disturbingly, however, media depictions of mental illness and sufferers are typically inaccurate and overwhelmingly negative (Alexander & Link, 2003; Wahl, 1992). Duckworth and colleagues (2003) randomly selected 1,740 American newspaper articles that mentioned schizophrenia or cancer between 1996 and 1997 and found that while only 1% of the articles cited cancer in an inaccurate metaphorical sense, there were 28% of such inaccurate citations for schizophrenia. Mehta and colleagues (2009) observed that public attitudes towards people with mental illness deteriorated during 1994–2003 in Britain, but especially in England and this situation was linked to the effect of adverse media reporting which took place over the time when changes to the Mental Health Act were widely debated and often reported in relation to the risk of violence posed by people with mental illness. The relatively more positive outlook in Scotland was linked to the early effect of the *See Me* campaign that was launched in Scotland in 2000.

Lalani and London (2006) observed what appeared to be an unquestioning acceptance in the British media of the 'rising toll of killings' as a result of community care for persons with mental illness. For instance, following the murder of Margaret Muller, an American woman found dead while jogging in Victoria Park in East London, the Daily Mail (February 21, 2003) published the headline, "400 care-in-the-community patients living by Murder Park". On discovering that a large number of care-in-the-community patients lived near the park, the police and the media automatically assumed that the victim was murdered by a deranged psychiatric patient living in the community.

On September 23, 2003, the former world heavyweight boxing champion Frank Bruno was admitted to a mental health unit in Essex. The Sun newspaper published a breaking news headline 'Bonkers Bruno Locked Up' that provoked a national outcry which forced the Sun to retract the headline. Suggestive headlines like this are pervasive as the print media consistently present the image of the dangerous, unstable, incurable mental patient. It is not uncommon in Britain to read the labels 'maniacs', 'schizos', 'psychos', and 'nutters' in the tabloid newspapers when stories are published about people with mental health problems. Even the traditionally more conventional broadsheet newspapers overwhelmingly tend to endorse this stereotype of people with mental illness as being potentially harmful to others, both in fictional and non-fictional representations (Philo, 1996).

A study found that people's attitudes towards those with mental illness markedly worsened directly after media reports of two violent attacks on prominent politicians by two persons with mental illness (Angermeyer & Schulze, 2001). Media portrayals fail to indicate that the percentage of violence that can be attributed to mental illness as a proportion of the general violence in the community is negligible (Monahan, 2009). When the media sensationalise the rare, but tragic events associated with someone having one of the serious mental disorders, they amplify fear while the significant majority who live full productive lives with these disorders are underrepresented.

Though the association between mental illness and violence, specifically schizophrenia, is confirmed epidemiologically (Arboleda-Florez, 1998), this seems to flow not so much through direct links of causality, but through a series of confounders such as co-morbid substance use and abuse (Davis, Uezato, Newell, & Frazier, 2008; Drake, McHugo, Xie, Fox, Packard, & Helmstetter, 2006). Unfortunately, one single case of violence is usually enough to undermine whatever gains patients with mental illness have made to be accepted back into the community. Even when reported conscientiously and accurately, this type of news provokes fear and apprehension and pushes the public to demand measures to prevent further crimes. Consequently, persons with mental illness, in general, bear the brunt of the impact as they are stereotyped because of the actions of the minority.

Two mass communication theories: cultivation theory and social cognitive theory (Stout, Villegas, & Jennings, 2004) provide the mechanisms by which the media influences mental illness stigma. The theories describe how the construction and perpetuation of mental illness stigma occur through the media's social construction of reality. While cultivation theory proposes that repeated exposure to consistent media messages shapes values and perceptions of reality to fit those presented in the media, social cognitive theory, on the other hand, proposes that, in addition to direct experience, individuals vicariously learn about appropriate behaviour and affective reactions through observation, particularly from media sources.

Workshops with journalists, in which information multipliers like the media are informed about the relationships between psychiatric illness and violence, and the potential consequences of careless and sensationalist reporting, have been reported to be helpful (Grausgruber et al., 2007). Thornton and Wahl (1996) administered two types of corrective information on subjects to investigate whether "corrective information" on mental illness could moderate the stigmatising effects of a newspaper article that described a murder committed by a person with mental illness. The first information addressed misconceptions about mental illness, for example, noting that violent behaviour is fairly rare among persons with mental illness while the second information highlighted the tendency of the media to present a distorted and prejudiced view of persons with mental illness. Results indicated that subjects who read either of the corrective information before reading the stigmatising newspaper article reported less fear and more acceptance of persons with mental illness than did subjects who did not receive the corrective information. This provided some evidence that corrective information may be effective in moderating the effect of negative reports and media coverage.

Nature and Symptom Presentation of Illness

People can also hold attitudes based on what they have experienced of the attitude object (Hugo, 2001). Thus, a major determinant of stigma is the behaviour of the person with mental illness and the associated disability. Illnesses that present in serious observable deformities or lesions like leprosy or extremely bizarre psychotic behaviours like schizophrenia are the most negatively perceived (Al-Krenawi et al., 2009; Marie & Miles, 2008; Mulatu, 1999). Symptom presentation is thus a significant determinant of stigma in sub-Saharan Africa, where symptoms of mental illness are mostly judged on behavioural grounds (Binitie, 1970). Manifest deviant behaviours attract mental illness labels and equate to psychiatric illness presentation in the involved person. Positive symptoms like disruptiveness, mainly from patients suffering from paranoid schizophrenia, can lead to the stereotype of dangerousness and unpredictability.

Hugo (2001) observed that the majority of mental health professionals' negative attitudes are informed by their experiences with people with mental health problems, many of which would be when the clients are experiencing crisis. A majority of the health workers report that it is difficult coping with persons with mental illness in the ward (Crisp, Gelder, Rix, & Meltzer, 2000; Oderinde et al., 2018). Two-thirds of nurses reported verbal or physical abuse in an Australian survey (Australian Nurses Federation, 2003). Fearing aggression, healthcare professionals who have faced violent experiences from persons with mental illness can develop a negative and avoidant attitude towards them which could lead to a biased view of the client's potential.

Penn and colleagues (1994) observed that the notion of previous symptomatology in the acute phase of schizophrenia was more stigmatising than a label alone. It may reinforce the stereotype of the recovered patient as unstable and, if the recovered person fails to deter the spread of such information, they may face rejection even if presenting with non-aberrant behaviour. Against such a backdrop, brief exposures during the acute phase of symptoms can be detrimental and can lead to increased social restrictiveness (Wallach, 2004).

Sometimes, serious mental illness like schizophrenia also manifests in negative symptoms such as alogia (poverty of speech), anhedonia (poverty of affect), avolition, and catatonia (motor abnormalities). These can constitute a serious hindrance to interaction with others and integration into society. Bell and colleagues (2008) report that more than half of pharmacy students in a cross-cultural study thought that patients with schizophrenia and severe depression were difficult to talk with, which may contribute to their receiving less medication counselling than patients with physical health disorders.

While aesthetics reflect what is attractive or pleasing to one's perceptions, in relation to stigma, it reflects the extent to which a characteristic elicits an instinctive and affective reaction of disgust (Jones et al., 1984). Thus, it constitutes a key distinguishing feature of persons with mental illness from the rest of the community especially in most of sub-Saharan Africa where the common appearance of persons with mental illness is that of unkempt vagrants (Atilola & Olayiwola, 2011; Ewhrudjakpor, 2010a). This is reinforced by a social representation of the body that is centred on beauty and well being (Goetz, Camargo, Bertoldo, & Justo, 2008). Associating mental illness with filth in the region is so normative that it has earned a place in the Igbo people's repertoire of anecdotes. For instance, to highlight the dirty appearance of motor mechanics in their professional work aprons, there is a local saying, *Ndi mekanik ekwerọzi ka-amara ndi bụ ndi ara* (With the way motor mechanics appear dirty, one is no longer able to distinguish who the real mad person is).

Diagnosis of Mental Illness and Psychiatric Hospitalisation

The complexity of mental illness stigma is such that diagnosis of mental illness and psychiatric hospitalisation in themselves can stigmatise

(Rao et al., 2009; Crabb et al., 2012). Torrey (1994) suggested that the stigma associated with a diagnosis is worse than dealing with the mental health problem itself. Similarly, the stigma that attends to accessing care for mental health problems has been considered to be a greater barrier to seeking help than the stigma attached to the condition itself (Rost, Smith, & Taylor, 1993). Openly discussing one's problems with mental health professionals can attract shame which could even lead to some patients being suicidal (Meltzer & colleagues, 2000). Patients try to contend with these through rejection of the psychiatric explanation of their problems (Sayre, 2000).

Although well-intentioned in its origins, the asylum mentality that saw to the sectioning of those with mental illness in isolated psychiatric hospitals contributed to social distance from them. It structurally helped to define them as different and led to their dislocation from their communities, loss of their community ties, friendships, and families. At a more systemic and academic level, institutionalisation meant the banishment of mental illness and psychiatry from the general stream of medicine, which helped to reinforce the idea that such patients were incurable (Arboleda-Flórez, 2001).

4 Consequences of the Stigma of Mental Illness

Social Exclusion

Stigma has the potential to impact on all aspects of life. It begets social exclusion. It strips people of their dignity and represents a major barrier to their effective rehabilitation and reintegration into society. It deprives sufferers of mental illness of their basic citizenship rights, happiness and sharing in the 'commonwealth' of life (Pilgrim, 2009;World Health Organization [WHO], 2001a). Moldovan (2007) notes that years after the introduction of the deinstitutionalisation policy, people with Serious and Persistent Mental Illness (SPMI) are still not well integrated into society. Sayce and Boradman (2003) observe that a major difficulty with the rehabilitation of people with mental illness is convincing members of the community such as employers or landlords that people can and do recover from mental illness. Stereotypes of violence and unpredictability inform the indisposition to share a neighbourhood with persons with mental illness (Department of Health, 2003; Wolff, Pathare & Craig, 1996). The case for deinstitutionalisation and care in the community is further not helped by the public notion that people with psychotic disorders commit particularly violent crimes and constitute a great danger for little children (Angermeyer & Matschinger, 2004).

As many as over four in five people in the case study of south-eastern Nigeria (Ikwuka, 2016) indicated that they would not let people who had recovered from mental illness take care of their children for a while. The findings compare with another Nigerian study of medical doctors where four in five would not accept a fully recovered psychiatric patient as a teacher of young children in a public school (Adewuya & Oguntade, 2007). As many as one-third of the respondents in the study also endorsed the social restrictiveness factor which expresses beliefs that people with mental illness are dangerous and are to be avoided or restricted.

In a study that investigated secondary school teachers' attitudes to mental illness in Ogun State, south-western Nigeria (Aghukwa, 2009b), 52% of teachers felt that persons with mental illness were unpredictable and they would therefore not want such persons to serve in the police force.

Over 68% of teachers would not want people who had been treated for mental illness to hold public jobs, 79% would not want them to serve as state ministers, 88% would not want them to be president, 84% would not want them to serve in the army, while 69% would not want them to serve as medical doctors. This echoes the finding from the pilot study for the World Psychiatric Association (WPA) Programme "Open the Doors", where 72% of the respondents believed that persons with schizophrenia could not work in regular jobs (Stuart & Arboleda-Flórez, 2001b).

Stigma can rob people with mental illness of opportunities for obtaining competitive employment, accessing services and living independently in a safe and comfortable home (Link & Phelan, 2006; Stuart, 2006). Stigmatising attitudes, especially of members of key groups such as employers, landlords and primary care physicians, can therefore be critical in the lives of people with mental illness. According to the 2017 UK National Health Service statistics, only 43% of people with mental health problems are in employment compared to 74% of the general population. The rate is as low as 8% for people with conditions such as schizophrenia. Pilgrim (2009) had submitted that people with mental illness are three times more likely to be unemployed than those with physical disabilities. The Citizens Advice Bureau, UK, reckons that this has more to do with the attitude of employers than lack of willingness on the part of the individual. While it is possible that mental illness could reduce motivation to fight for a job, a study by Rethink Mental Illness (Scott, 2017) found that two-thirds of people with mental illness who are unemployed are either looking for work or want to work.

The study found that 68% of employers would worry that someone with a severe mental illness wouldn't fit in with the team. Eighty-three per cent would worry that someone with severe mental illness wouldn't be able to cope with the demands of the job while 74% would worry that such staff would require lots of time off. Yet, the 'mentally ill' label does not necessarily mean that someone cannot cope with work, won't fit in, or will require lots of time off. Moreover, the workplace should be able to provide the flexibility and understanding that support required adjustments. Disturbingly, over half of the employers of labour surveyed in the study admitted lacking the capacity to support someone with a severe mental health condition at work. Indeed, the Citizens Advice Bureau reported that persons with mental illness who have jobs end up leaving because their employers convince them instead that they are unable to cope.

People with mental illness can fear losing their job where they are employed. Some believe that they were dismissed or denied employment because of their condition (Putman, 2008). In the report by Scott (2017), Denise who suffers from mental illness recounts, "I've been affected by mental illness since I was 16 years old but was diagnosed with bipolar when I was 25. Despite my mental health condition, I worked as a mental health nurse all my life until 2011. I became physically unwell in 2011 with spinal problems and was forced to leave my job. Being off work for a long period of time has really knocked my confidence, but when I've felt better I've been able to go for job interviews. It's always a dilemma as to whether I should disclose the fact that I have bipolar or not. It feels like a risk, which it shouldn't be, and unfortunately I have experienced stigma when I have disclosed .... I had a job offer withdrawn at the last minute when I told them about my condition. It feels like I'm stuck between a rock and a hard place – a benefits system and the workplace, neither of which understand mental illness."

In a study by Dunn (1991), Jo, a mental health service user relayed her experiences at work. When she told her boss that she had to see a psychiatrist, "... his reaction said it all. As soon as mental illness is mentioned, people literally back away from you." At the workplace, employees with mental illness note that colleagues can be unsupportive, making snide remarks and feeling that they should do more to 'make up' for the fact that they have an illness (Warner, 2002). They can be advised to lower their expectations for a productive life and denied insurance coverage (Björkman, Angelman & Jönsson, 2008; Wahl, 1999). Social exclusion is thus a complicated and often cyclical process; limited access to one service can have a knock-on effect on others. For instance, restricted use of education and training opportunities can sustain unemployment, leading to more dependency on benefit, which deepens a person's exclusion, causing further decline in their health and quality of life.

The World Health Organisation highlights the pervasive role of mental health stigma in society with regard to suffering, disability, poverty, alcohol misuse, drug abuse, homelessness, or excessive institutionalisation (WHO, 2001a). Stigmatisation also damages inter-personal relationships including friendships, marriage and family relations (Fabrega, 2001; Kermode et al., 2009; Kung, 2003; Wahl & Harman, 1989). Discrimination is evident in every area of life, particularly for those suffering from psychosis and drug dependence (Rao et al., 2009).

In a study by Crawford and Brown (2002), a patient with schizophrenia shares her telling experiences whereby her actions (which should normally have been considered on their merits) were interpreted from the perspective of her mental illness. " ... [S]o you're sat at home on high tranquillisers. [Laughter] You try and go out up the club for a drink, and you have one drink with your medication and you're sat in the pub like this. [Laughter] I think everyone thought I was a junky... Because I'd go in the pub and have one drink, and I'd be all floaty and happy. And they'd say, 'Hey, she is off her head.' It is very hard to live with it, especially in a small community, because everyone knows everyone else's business." This submission also underscores the observation that there is a lack of confidentiality and the possibility of interference with intimate problems in small closed systems (Levav et al., 2004; Papadopoulos et al., 2002). Institutional stigmatisation can equally occur whereby the idea that 'mad people' are also being treated in the community facility is abhorrent to some people such as people living in the neighbourhood and some health staff (Gater, Jordanova, Maric, & Alikaj, 2005).

With the recognition that no single individual is self-sufficient, the basic principle of the closely-knit kinship system in the mostly communalistic sub-Saharan African cultures is that of co-prosperity. This is captured in the maxim *onye aghala nwanne ya* (Be your brother's keeper) of the Igbo of south-eastern Nigeria. This system acts as the economic, social and medical units where strong members lend support to the weak (Onwuejeogwu, 1986). Such a pro-community care philosophy is expected to facilitate the deinstitutionalisation and community approach of contemporary mental healthcare. It is thus incongruous that close to a third of the population (29.8%) in the case study of south-eastern Nigerian (Ikwuka, 2016) opposed community care.

The contradiction in attitude is reinforced by the fact that although 96.7% and 70.2% of respondents in the study expressed benevolent and pro-community care views, respectively, 71.4% considered such a move very risky. An equally very high percentage (85.7%) endorsed social distance from people with mental illness at primary (e.g. marriage) and even secondary (e.g. sharing neighbourhood) (52.4%) levels of relationship. This compares with a study of the Nigerian public where close to two-thirds (64.6%) admitted they could not live with, or get married to, someone with mental illness (Aina, Oshodi, Erinfolami, Adeyemi, & Suleiman, 2015). This pits practice against principle and could be a reflection of the NIMBY (not in my backyard) attitude, whereby people could support an ideology due to the social desirability factor but would not be open to the experience in practice due to an entrenched aversion to the attitude object (Cowan, 2003; Leff & Warner, 2006).

It reflects the contradiction in the findings of Komiti and colleagues (2006) where the majority of participants (over 70%) believed that people in their respective communities would gossip about a person who had a mental illness and that many would be wary of someone who had been hospitalised for a mental illness, yet most respondents believed that their respective communities would be supportive and caring towards someone with a mental illness. In a survey of mental health service providers in the UK National Health Service (NHS) and the voluntary sector, Repper and colleagues (1997) found that two-thirds had experienced NIMBY campaigns. The social desirability factor will be heightened in communitarian societies where solidarity with the disabled is normative of the social value system.

An anti-community care stance could also be indicative of the stress that the home care of people with mental illness brings to families including: day-to-day practical constraints in social and work life, psychological distress engendered by the illness, problems in intra-family relationships, severe economic hardships and heightened associative stigma (Corrigan, Druss, Perlick, 2014; Wahl & Harman, 1989). These could all have more impact in an intrusive communitarian culture. Corroborating this, Perlick and colleagues (2004) found that greater family perceptions of devaluation, and discrimination of both persons with the illness and their family members, were associated with higher levels of burden.

However, given that the solidarity of communitarian societies has been acclaimed as compensating for the deficient mental health infrastructure in these societies (Harrison et al., 2001; Hopper & Wanderling, 2000), it is disturbing that the cohesive network is potentially undermined by an anti-community care attitude, the domestic challenges notwithstanding. This fear is already being confirmed in the finding of a Nigerian study which looked at long-term social outcomes among a group of persons with schizophrenia who were receiving outpatient care. Contrary to the expectation that traditional family networks and supports would buffer these patients against drifting down in socio-economic status, they continued to experience severe social disabilities in multiple domains (Gureje & Bamidele, 1999).

Yet, deinstitutionalisation has implications for how the process of stigma may operate in practice. In the study by Crawford and Brown (2002), a mental health worker reports: "Sometimes we see people here [at the clinic] rather than at home, because they actually don't want us visiting at home in case the neighbours see. So we make arrangements for them to come here. So they don't want you coming looking like someone from a mental health facility …. Sometimes if you've got two in the same street, I'd perhaps leave my car round the corner and walk round." One of the healthcare staff in the study suggested that mental health service paraphernalia such as a briefcase, diary, and pen badges should all be concealed as such confidentiality helps to keep stigma at bay to some extent. Even mail can be suggestive in appearance if it has mental hospital postmark on it. One of the health workers observed: "[Gossip] … goes like wildfire … you know with local people, neighbours, letters you get through the post … they've got the name of the hospital …. The postman, the temporary ones, as well … in villages ….."

The good intentions of the deinstitutionalisation policies notwithstanding, when adequate community systems to house those with mental illness and provide for their successful reintegration into the community are lacking; stigma is worsened when persons with mental illness are observed roaming the high streets, loitering in town squares, shopping centres or markets, or being destitute homeless vagrants (Arboleda-Flórez, 2001). Beyond entering into clients' subjective worlds therefore, professionals will have to confront the everyday problems with living which clients face. As Wainer and Chesters (2000) indicate, a successful deinstitutionalisation process would thus entail mental healthcare becoming more integrated; involving helping clients to have enough to live on, to have a home, a job, relationships and friends, and to be free from violence and stigma.

Structural Discrimination

Structural stigma reflects policies of private and public institutions that intentionally or unintentionally restrict opportunities for people with mental illness. Some inequities represented by system-level barriers are attributed to this process, for example, state legislation that limits the civil rights of people with mental illness. Studies examining state legislation in the 1980s (Burton, 1990) and 1990s (Hemmens, Miller, Burton, & Milner, 2002) indicated that as many as 20 states in the US restricted voting, jury duty, elective office, parenting, and marriage rights because of mental illness. Some of the restrictions were informed by the stigmatising beliefs that people with mental illness are not capable of being full citizens or family members (Pelletier, Davidson, Roelandt, & Daumerie, 2009).

Attitudes also influence policy decisions regarding persons with mental illness in terms of their rights (Levey & Howells, 1994) and planning of psychiatric services (Mino, Kodera, & Bebbington, 1990). Research indicates that endorsing stigma is inversely related to resource allocation. People who endorsed the idea that people are to blame for their mental illness were less likely to provide more money to mental health programmes in a government fund allocation task (Corrigan, Watson, Warpinski, & Gracia, 2004b). Legislators who endorse stereotypes of persons with mental illness can block funding for mental health services that may promote independent living and recovery goals (Corrigan et al., 2004b).

In the Report on Mental Health issued by the US Surgeon General, the stigma of mental illness was noted for reduced levels of service funding (U.S. Department of Health and Human Services, 1999). In Canada, mental health research commands less than 5% of all the health research budgets, yet mental illness directly affects 20% of Canadians (Canadian Alliance on Mental Illness and Mental Health, 2000). In spite of being a leading cause of disability, it is observed that mental health receives the least funding in the health budgets of many developing countries. Often, less than 1% of expenditure on health is made on services for psychiatric conditions in African countries (Kleinman, 2009). A high premium is placed on infectious disease and maternal and child health, as evidenced by high budgetary allocations to these sectors in comparison to mental health services (Ayorinde, Gureje, & Lawal, 2004; Gureje, 2003). Relative to other illnesses, schizophrenia receives low levels of funding for research, and treatment facilities for schizophrenia tend to be located in isolated settings or disadvantaged neighbourhoods (Link, Yang, Phelan, & Collins, 2004).

People with mental disorders are more likely to be uninsured or underinsured than the general population (Garfield, Zuvekas, Lave, & Donohue, 2011). Health insurance companies openly discriminate against persons who acknowledge that they have had a mental health problem. Companies issuing life insurance and income protection policies make the continuation of payments an ordeal for people suffering a temporary disability caused by mental health conditions such as anxiety or depression with many patients seeing their payments denied or their policies discontinued (Arboleda-Flórez, 2001). Persistent structural stigma, such as insurance barriers and inadequate systems of community support stall effective efforts to prevent or treat mental illness and leads to negative socio-economic consequences such as the loss of a productive workforce (Keusch, Wilentz, & Kleinman, 2006; Link & Phelan, 2006; Stuart, 2005).

Structural discrimination can also take place with regard to legal provision as well as the interpretation and administration of laws (Gutierrez-Lobos, 2002). The criminalisation of mental illness occurs when people with mental health problems are dealt with by the police, courts and jails, instead of the mental health system (Watson, Corrigan, & Ottati, 2004). Persons with mental illness spend more time in incarceration compared with non-sufferers (Steadman, McCarty, & Morrissey, 1989). They are more likely to be accused falsely of violent crimes (Sosowsky, 1980; Steadman, 1981) leading to their higher arrest rates (Goodman, 1992; Raymond, 1991) even when they are actually more likely to be victims.

Though nearly half of service users had been verbally or physically harassed in public because of their mental illness (Read & Baker, 1996), many could be denied justice should they seek redress as they are often not seen as credible witnesses and prosecutions are frequently dropped (Women against Rape/Legal Action for Women, 1995). A leading Nigerian newspaper *The Punch* reported an incident where a young man sexually violated female residents of a mental health facility in Lagos state. The young man was charged and taken to court, but the prosecution could not proffer rape charges against him "due to the mental health status of the victim. A case of breaching public peace was rather preferred" (Adesomoju, 2013).

Specific policy measures may also fuel already fearful and intolerant public attitudes towards people with mental illness. In response to high-profile but isolated incidents in which vulnerable people with mental health problems have taken the lives of others, there was a suggestion that the UK government considered a review of community mental healthcare apparently to "maintain the safety of the public" (Thomson & Sylvester, 1998). To "clean up the streets", a state government in south-western Nigeria gathered some destitute vagrant sufferers of psychosis ('mad people'), herded them into a truck, and 'deported' them to their states of origin in the eastern part of the same country, against their constitutional right of abode in any part of the country. There, they were abandoned, and some reportedly died after some days (Okpi, 2013). Similarly, a state government in south-southern part of Nigeria quarantined such 'mad people' and engaged the services of native doctors to manage their decline (Ewhrudjakpor, 2009).

Such situations are not helped by the lack of expeditious enactment of enabling laws in Nigeria, as exemplified in the delayed passing into law of the mental health bill proposed by the Association of Nigerian Psychiatrists. The existing legislation dates back to a British colonial law of 1916 that was later revised as the Lunacy Act in 1958, a designation so telling of mental illness stigma. Most successful initiatives recognise the role of legislation as a tool against stigma and discrimination (Idoko, 2013). Mental health legislation should be made more flexible and pertinent to contemporary mental health policies and the realities of the mental health system.

Increased Burden of Disease

Stigma has been described as a "second illness" (Finzen, 1996). As earlier noted, the damaging impact has been compared to and considered arguably worse than that of the devastating symptoms. Thus, stigma constitutes double jeopardy for sufferers. Granted that stigma can make some people with mental illness more determined to succeed, the overwhelming negative impacts can persist despite psychiatric treatment and recovery.

Stigma results in both short and long-term personal distress for affected people. It can have a significant negative impact on the psychosocial functioning of people with mental illnesses through both experienced and anticipated discrimination. Stigma consciousness (anticipated stigma) is where individuals fear being categorised within a stigmatised group because they are perceived as carrying certain traits, for instance, they fear being labelled 'mentally ill' which is socially stigmatised (Pinel, 1999). In the absence of overt discrimination, they may anticipate stigmatising responses at work and in relationships and become preoccupied with concealing their status. This can exacerbate paranoid symptoms for people with serious mental illness, for example, schizophrenia.

Perceived stigma leads to significant loss of self-esteem and self-efficacy, depression, limiting of social and occupational functioning, withdrawal and reduced trust in others (Corrigan, 2004; Link, Struening, Neese-Todd, Asmussen, & Phelan, 2001; Perlick et al., 2001). Stigma can generate emotional feelings of fear, anxiety, anger, hurt, sadness, discouragement, isolation, guilt and embarrassment (Dinos, Stevens, Serfaty, Weich, & King, 2004; Wahl, 1999). It may increase the environmental stress of persons with mental illness and decrease their ability to cope (Link, 1982).

Failed by the state and abandoned by overwhelmed families, many persons with serious mental disorders in Nigeria and most of sub-Saharan Africa live as vagrants on the streets and in open market squares where they feed from waste bins and are exposed to the extremes of weather without shelter. Ironically, the negligent society has a supposed wisdom in an Igbo proverb, *Ara ọụrụ ahia, adighi agwọ ya agwọ* (Once madness [a mad person] strays into the market square, it [he/she] becomes irremediable). This presupposes the presence of some mysterious forces in the market square that exacerbate symptoms. Yet, it is easily explainable that exposure to the elements and the harsh living conditions are factors that would more likely exacerbate and perpetuate symptoms.

Almost half of the service users surveyed by Read and Baker (1996) had been verbally or physically harassed in public because of their mental illness. In the study by Crawford and Brown (2002), a patient with schizophrenia recounts the ordeal of labelling: "I came back from the toilet once and this bloke making a nice comment about how I looked. Then this other bloke went, 'Oh no, she's a nutter, you don't want to go there!' and I heard them say it, and I said, 'Oh, I'm a nutter am I?' I said. 'Well, how come I can have a serious conversation with you then?' I've done this, I've done that. I really pointed him up on it, what it was really like to be labelled a nutter. He was so sorry afterwards, and he comes over and talks to me now. It's the fear of the unknown. Once you get a label." Indeed, the 'fear of the unknown' aptly underscores the burden of living with mental illness both in terms of the symptoms and the stigma.

Impedance of Help-Seeking

The prejudice and discrimination that characterise the stigma of mental illness significantly contribute to the disconnect between effective treatments and care-seeking (Corrigan et al., 2014). The unwanted repercussions of mental health stigma, such as anticipated and experienced discrimination, and poor treatment both personally and professionally, have all been linked to the taboo of help-seeking for mental health problems globally (Yoshimura, Bakolis, & Henderson, 2018). Individuals who do not seek help fear the judgement and persecution of public opinion should they be found in a scenario that does not conform to socially accepted views of health and wellbeing (Corrigan & Shapiro, 2010; Lucksted & Drapalski, 2015).

Research underscores how stigma serves as a barrier to help-seeking for children (Adler & Wahl, 1998), adolescents (Chandra & Minkovitz, 2007), adults (Vogel, Wade, & Hackler, 2007), and elders (Graham et al., 2003). Stigma impacts care seeking at personal, provider, and system levels. Stigma and discrimination can impede access to care at institutional, community and individual levels in the following ways: institutional through legislation, funding, and availability of services (Corrigan et al., 2004b); community through public attitudes and behaviours (Evans-Lacko, Baum, Danis, Biddle, & Goold, 2012), and individual through self-stigmatisation and feelings of shame in seeking help (Rüsch et al., 2009).

Stigma underlies the shame and secrecy associated with suffering from mental illness, and the reluctance to self-disclose which inhibits access to care as sufferers are wary of how others will view them once they disclose their disorder (Byrne, 2000; Dinos et al., 2004; Tanaka, Ogawa, Inadomi, Kikuchi & Ohta, 2003). Similarly, they attempt to avoid the unfair discrimination and loss of opportunity that comes with stigmatising labels by avoiding going to clinics or interacting with mental health providers with whom the prejudice is associated (Corrigan, 2004). Patients who are seen by non-psychiatric health workers in general health facilities are apprehensive of referral to psychiatrists or other mental health professionals (Hartley, Korsea, Bird, & Agger, 1998; Regier et al., 1993). This arises in most circumstances for reasons that include patients feeling more comfortable with non-psychiatric workers in general health facilities and the desire to avoid being labelled 'mentally ill'.

In a study of a rural Australian community (Fuller, Edwards, Procter, & Moss, 2000), the authors report that every person they interviewed concluded that mental health problems were associated with a high degree of stigma, and many suggested that they were associated with fear. A social worker in the study reported that "... a lot of people won't come in (for treatment) because...mental health (has) got that stigma ... you know, I'm not a nut case ..." and according to a telephone counsellor in the study: "... some are shocked when you ... try to give them a referral to a mental health service. Because they may think that's only for weirdos, people who are mad." A mental health consumer and advocate in the study similarly declared that "... because of the stigma attached to mental illness ... the last thing you want to do is to go into the system and seek help."

The conventional understanding of mental health problems as implying irremediable insanity leads to a fear about what happens to people who become clients within the mental healthcare system. The telephone counsellor further stated: "... [people] see mental health as like the one step on from ... [the asylum] ... like all the people in the white coats. 'I don't need that sort of thing.'" The implication is that, even when people do recognise their distress, they may avoid formal mental health services, not perceiving them as an appropriate source of help. Owing to stigma, some would still not seek help even when the situation has become critical. The South African Federation of Mental Health (2011) revealed that South Africans would rather die than admit to mental illness.

Stigma is a powerful inhibitive factor for help-seeking even for battle-hardened soldiers. Over 3000 military staff from the US Army or Marine Corps units that had served combat duty in Iraq or Afghanistan were anonymously surveyed three to four months after their return. They were assessed for depression, anxiety, or post-traumatic stress disorder (PTSD). The majority of the affected soldiers (60–77%) did not seek mental healthcare mostly due to concerns about possible stigmatisation (Hoge et al., 2004).

It has also been argued that self-stigma is a much more potent stigma that may directly inhibit help-seeking since the individual perceives the act of seeking professional help for distress as a threat to their self-worth and as a weakness of character (Vogel & Wade, 2009). Families and relatives, who are stigmatised by association, could hide ill relatives and not talk about their condition, thus practically foreclosing access to care. Associative stigma could add to the burden of care which could lead to extreme measures such as child abuse, neglect or abandonment with a report alleging that some mothers of children with intellectual disabilities had considered doing away with their children in Nigeria (Abasiubong, Obembe, & Ekpo, 2006).

Thus, stigma leads to non-utilisation, underutilisation or delay in the utilisation of mental health services, living in denial of mental health problems and early termination of mental health treatment. Delay in seeking medical treatment at the onset of illness results in symptoms being aggravated as patients try to cope on their own and the family is frightened of the consequences of releasing this information (Tanaka et al., 2003). Studying Arab clients in mental health settings, Al-Krenawi and Graham (2000) noted that stigma might have a particularly gendered implication with the potential damage that mental health help-seeking could cause to present and future marital prospects of females, including the possibility of divorce or the husband taking on a second polygamous wife.

Over 70% of Arab American women reported feelings of shame associated with seeking formal social services, and almost this number, too, reported embarrassment associated with reporting their problem to people outside of their family (Al-Krenawi, Graham, Al-Bedah, Kadri, & Sehwail, 2009). On the other hand, men may associate formal help-seeking with a diminishment of their masculinity and abilities to be strong providers and family leaders (see Chapter 7, Culture of Self Reliance).

Impedance of Treatment and Recovery

Stigma is arguably the most significant obstacle to appropriate treatment, rehabilitation, and recovery, and to the development of effective care and treatment for those suffering from mental illness (Bell et al., 2008; Pitre, Stewart, Adams, Bedard, & Landry, 2007; Sartorius, 2002). It causes delays in diagnosis (Corrigan, Green, Lundin, Kubiak, & Penn, 2001) and has been identified as a primary obstacle to progress in mental illness prevention and research (Schomerus & Angermeyer, 2008;

Thornicroft, 2008). People with mental illness receive less medical attention than others (Druss et al., 2001). The fear of 'madness' begets social distancing which undermines the therapeutic efforts of service users and professionals, reducing their ability to provide effective care (Foskett, Marriott, & Wilson-Rudd, 2004).

Using data from the 1990 National Co-morbidity Survey in the US, Wang, Demler, and Kessler (2002) estimated that only 20% of individuals with serious mental illnesses treated in general medical settings, and 45.7% of those treated in speciality mental health settings, received adequate treatment for their conditions. Stigma, and its attendant discrimination, stall recovery, and reintegration following a period of illness, and result in lost opportunities for fuller participation in life (Corrigan et al., 2001). A major obstacle to the success of programmes such as the Supported Education Programme (SEP) for adults with schizophrenia, which helps in the rehabilitation of persons with mental illness, is the negative stigmatising attitudes of the professionals responsible for the daily running of the programmes towards psychiatric disorders and persons with mental illness (Corrigan et al., 2004a).

In a national survey of New Zealand, service users reported discrimination in mental health services which included: failure to provide appropriate services and information, providing disrespectful or inappropriate treatment, failing to respect information from family members, and perpetuating negative stereotypes. They equally reported physical abuse, being talked about rather than to, feeling degraded, or being put down, and ridiculed. Some felt abuse was often very subtle and specific to an individual staff member while others reported it as overt and endemic (The Mental Health Foundation of New Zealand, 2003).

Patients with mental illness who perceive devaluation or rejection by others have been shown to have worse outcomes (Link, Struening, Rahav, Phelan, & Nuttbrock, 1997). For instance, fear of stigma and lack of understanding of puerperal psychosis by families and healthcare professionals were linked to the finding that women with a severe psychiatric disorder had a 70-fold increased risk of committing postnatal suicide and that mothers with mental illness who kill their children do so often as an extension of suicide (Appleby, Mortensen, & Faragher, 1998; Craig, 2004; Spinelli, 2004). Consistent with the diathesis-stress model of schizophrenia, heightened environmental stressors such as job loss, rejection by suitors etc. associated with being stigmatised might equally contribute to relapse.

Persistent structural stigma, such as insurance barriers and inadequate systems of support, lead to degeneration of poorly treated disease, additional disability, injury, or even death (Link & Phelan, 2006; Stuart, 2005). Limited funding and provider shortages hamper access to care in community mental health settings, particularly in poor and rural areas, especially for people with more disabling diagnoses such as schizophrenia and bipolar disorder (Hough, Willging, Altschul, & Adelsheim, 2011). Stigma can worsen symptoms and increase the risk of co-morbid physical disease (Chapman, Perry, & Strine, 2005). The rejecting attitudes of the health workers, on the other hand, lead to their inability to detect co-morbid physical illnesses in psychiatric patients, and where they are detected, the patients are reluctantly and inappropriately cared for (Aghukwa, 2009a).

Stigma could lead to medication non-compliance (Barney, Griffiths, Jorm, & Christensen, 2006; Haghighat, 2001) and affect psychiatric treatment adherence (Sirey et al., 2001). Mkize and Uys (2004) reported how a client defaulted in treatment because of his siblings' negative reference to his treatment: "Take your tablets for madness." A study of pathways to psychiatric care in Eastern Europe (Gater, Jordanova, Maric, & Alikaj, 2005) found a preference for 'mild' medicines (such as sedatives or hypnotics) which are less taboo to 'strong' medicines (such as antidepressants or antipsychotics) with connotations of severe mental illness.

5   Pervasiveness of Stigma

The Developing World

Earlier studies had suggested that stigmatising attitudes towards persons with mental illness are less evident in more traditionalist (non-Western) societies (Carothers, 1948; Cheetham & Rzadkowolski, 1980; Fabrega, 1991). Cooper and Sartorius (1977) noted a suggestion that social representation of mental diseases in such societies, with supposedly less differentiation between mental and physical illnesses, as well as a religious dimension in the conceptualisation of mental illness have a preventive effect on stigmatisation. Disputing this claim, however, a leading Nigerian psychiatrist and scholar, Gureje (2007), reported that it borders on the exotic, and reflects an erroneous tendency to present such societies as some sort of El Dorado where, unlike in 'civilised communities', no distinction is made between the sane and the insane, with everybody living together in blissful happiness. He went further to articulate the common knowledge that, in Africa, for instance, sufferers are socially alienated and abused as a result of their illness, often along with their families. Disaffiliated families sometimes abandon and disown their sick members because of societal stigma and shame.

A study of Moroccan families of patients with schizophrenia found that most of the families suffer from stigma and discrimination, with a total of 86.7% reporting that they have hard lives because of the illness, and 72% reporting psychological suffering caused by sleep and relationship disturbances and a poor quality of life (Kadri, Manoudi, Berrada, & Moussaoui, 2004). An Ethiopian survey revealed a widespread experience of stigma suffered by people with mental illness with three-quarters of their family members also experiencing stigma (Shibre et al., 2001). Only a quarter of a Malawian study sample believed that mental illness could be treated outside of the hospital setting (Crabb et al., 2012).

Negative attitudes towards people with mental illness are prevalent in Nigerian communities. A seminal work (Gureje, Lasebikan, Ephraim-Oluwanuga, Olley, & Kola, 2005), which investigated community knowledge of and attitudes towards mental illness in south-western

Nigeria, found that most of the respondents thought that people with mental illness were mentally retarded, a public nuisance, dangerous because of their violent behaviour and could not be treated outside the hospital. Only about a quarter thought that persons with mental illness could work in regular jobs. The five most endorsed personal attributes of persons with mental illness in a survey of doctors in the same southwestern Nigeria included: unpredictable, dangerous, lacking self-control, aggressive, and dependent. A study of the same region also found pessimism of prognosis, with only 9% of doctors believing that mental illness could be cured (Adewuya & Oguntade, 2007).

Eighty-one per cent of schizophrenia sufferers studied in Lagos, southwestern Nigeria, have been discriminated against and avoided by people who found out they had schizophrenia, 71% experienced unfair treatment from family members, 63% from friends, 32% from society, 29% from intimate relationships, and 39% in personal safety (Adeosun, Adegbohun, Jeje & Adewumi, 2013). More than a third of healthcare providers surveyed in south-southern Nigeria indicated that they would indeed shun or outrightly reject family members suffering from mental illness (Ewhrudjakpor, 2009). A study of the senior medical staff of a University Teaching Hospital in the same south-southern Nigeria (Ukpong & Abasiubong, 2010) revealed strong authoritarian and socially restrictive attitudes towards patients with mental illness.

Seventy-eight per cent of respondents in the study disagreed with the view that large mental hospitals are an outdated means of treating people with mental illness, 75% thought there is something about persons with mental illness that makes it easy to differentiate them from 'normal people', 69.2% disagreed with the view that less emphasis should be placed on protecting the public from them, 62% thought that persons with mental illness needed the same kind of control as children, 62% believed that a person should be hospitalised once he or she displayed signs of mental illness, 40% disagreed that mental illness was like any other illness while 16.3% believed that custodial care under lock and key was the best way to handle mental health patients.

In addition, 82.7% believed that persons with mental illness should lose their human rights, 50% disagreed with the suggestion that women who were once patients in a mental hospital could be trusted as babysitters, 32.7% believed that persons with mental illness should not be given any responsibility, 27.0% believed that anyone with a history of mental illness should be excluded from taking public office and 22.1% would not like to live next door to someone who suffers from mental illness. The majority of journalists (97%) and nurses (89%) in a comparative study of the same south-southern Nigeria believed that people with mental illness are dangerous, violent and should not be married (Abasiubong, Ekott, & Bassey, 2007). Most respondents in a study of non-mental health workers in north-eastern Nigeria reported that they would keep a social distance from people with mental illness because they are dangerous (Oderinde et al., 2018).

Pervasive negative attitudes were evident in the case study of south-eastern Nigeria (Ikwuka, 2016) with more than half of all the surveyed demographic groups (nurses 56.6%, teachers 79.0%, students 89.4% and the general public 87.6%) demonstrating authoritarian attitudes which see a clear difference between persons with mental illness and others and proposes immediate hospitalisation for them. A highly significant percentage of all the demographic groups desired social distance from persons cured of mental illness at closer levels of association; nurses (79.3%), teachers (87.6%), students (88.2%), and the general public (89.0%). Over a third of the nurses (35.4%) and more than half of those in the non-nursing occupational groups (teachers 60.9%, students 59.2%, the general public 60.6%) also desired social distance from people cured of mental illness at secondary (less intimate) levels of association. Eighty-two per cent of the respondents would not marry someone who had recovered from mental illness, 85% would not agree to such a person babysitting their child, and 76% would not accept them as a house-help.

Seventy-nine per cent of the respondents would not share secrets with people who have been cured of mental illness, 77.4% would not have them as sureties or witnesses, while 54.4% would not seek their advice on sundry issues. Seventy-one per cent would neither accept to be driven in a car by someone who has been cured of mental illness, nor employ such persons as security guards, while 56.4% would not do business with them. Seventy per cent would not argue with people that have been cured of mental illness, 40% would not be close friends with them, 31% would not play or share jokes with them, while 45.4% would not share belongings with them. Twenty-six per cent would not live in the same house with such persons, while 53.4% would not live in the same compound with them. Seventy-eight per cent would not receive an injection from a nurse who had been cured of mental illness, and 56.4% would not agree to such persons barbing or doing their hair.

About a third of all the groups (teachers 41.0%, students 40.1%, general public 35.2%) except nurses (16.2%) also endorsed the social restriction of persons with mental illness. Again, with the exception of the nurses (9.0%), over a third of teachers (44.7%) and the general public (36.1%), with 27.8% of students, demonstrated opposition to their care in the community (deinstitutionalisation). Almost all those surveyed (94.7%) saw people with mental illness as different to others while 78.9% reckoned that mental illness is unlike any other illness. Ninety-two per cent felt that anybody who displayed signs of mental illness should be hospitalised immediately, with 30.2% suggesting that they should be locked away. Forty-seven per cent of the respondents thought that people with mental illness were a burden the society. As many as 27.4% believed that they have no human rights. Fifty-one per cent thought that they should not be given responsibility, while 48.3% felt that they should not serve in public office. Sixty-five per cent believed that they were as needy and dependent as children. Considering that the degree of social distance established by the study was as desired from those already cured of mental illness, it should be expected that those still living with the condition would experience even greater negative attitudes.

Marriage prospects, fear of rejection by neighbours, and the need to hide the illness from others were among the additional concerns of people with schizophrenia and their caregivers in India (Thara & Srinivasan, 2000). In the Erwadi tragedy in South India in 2001, more than 20 persons with mental illness were burnt to death when a fire swept one of the treatment shelters near the healing mosque where they were chained to their beds (Murthy, 2001). Therefore, the findings add to the refutation of the earlier submissions that had claimed that non-Western traditionalist and borderline societies appeared to be immune to stigmatising attitudes towards people with mental illness. The earlier reports may have been due to a paucity of research rather than suggesting that people in the region held more receptive attitudes towards mental illness.

The Developed World

Surveys of North America and Western Europe indicate that stigma is a major concern in the community. A comparison of datasets from the 1950 national survey with a 1996 survey did not demonstrate a significant change in the stigmatising attitudes of the American public who believe that people who experience psychosis are dangerous (Phelan, Link, Stueve, & Pescosolido, 2000). Using similar questions and similarly designed studies, 77% of respondents in Germany (Gaebel, Baumann, Witte, & Zaeske, 2002) and 75% in Canada (Stuart & Arbodela-Flórez, 2001b) would be unwilling to have someone suffering from drug or alcohol dependency, schizophrenia, or depression marry a family member.

Offensive newspaper and poster advertisements were once published in America for a film titled *Crazy People.* They included a picture of a cracked egg with hands and arms and the caption, "Warning: Crazy people are coming" (Wahl, 1995). A mental health 'survivor', in a Canadian survey, reported: "I have to lie to my landlord to get a place to live, like tell him you are on disability, if it is not visible or physical, they don't take you. Even slumlords won't take you because they don't want psychiatrically ill people living in their buildings." 'Survivors' in the study reported that they felt ignored, avoided, or treated without respect and sensitivity (People Advocating for Change through Empowerment [P.A.C.E.] Report, 1996).

Sixty-seven per cent of respondents in a study of Australia (Griffiths et al., 2006) thought that people with chronic schizophrenia are unpredictable, while a third of consumers with mental health problems surveyed in New Zealand, reported having been discriminated against by mental health services (The Mental Health Foundation of New Zealand, 2003). In Italy, where psychiatry has a long history of community treatments, a study conducted ten years after the promulgation of the 1978 psychiatric reform law found that the general public held negative attitudes towards those with mental illness (Kemali, Maj, Veltro, Crepet, & Lobrace, 1989). A study of Greek public attitudes towards persons with mental illness found a direct association of schizophrenia with criminality (Economou, Gramandani, Richardson, & Stefanis, 2005), while a large-scale representative national survey of the British adult population found pervasive negative opinions that exaggerated the disabilities of mental illness (Crisp, Gelder, Rix, Meltzer, & Rowlands, 2000).

In September 2013, the supermarket chains Tesco and Asda in the UK were forced to apologise following a public outcry against their stereotypical association of mental illness with the weird ghosts of Halloween. Asda had produced a 'mental patient fancy dress costume' with the catchphrase "Everyone will be running away from you in fear in this mental patient fancy dress." Tesco equally displayed a costume called 'Psycho Ward'. Earlier, in March 2006, the BBC and other media reported the public outcry against the statue of Prime Minister Winston Churchill in a straitjacket which was commissioned by the mental health charity *Rethink* and unveiled in the Norwich area to draw attention to and stamp out the stigma surrounding mental health. Churchill was highlighted because, despite dealing with the symptoms of manic depression throughout his life, he was able to become Prime Minister, lead the country during World War II and was voted "The Greatest Briton" in a national poll. But the public, including the politician's family and World War II veterans, interpreted the concept as 'distasteful', 'absurd' and 'pathetic' and their complaints eventually led to the removal of the sculpture.

A similar scenario was recorded in China where a coffee shop run by people with mental health problems was forced to shut down due to the protests of the local community (Song, Chang, Shih, Lin, & Yang, 2005). Another Chinese study noted that persons with mental illness are always seen as potential sources of social instability because it is feared that they are volatile (Park, Xiao, Worth, & Park, 2005). Associative stigma is equally rife in the Chinese collectivist culture where mental illness is highly stigmatising for the whole family, not just the afflicted individual. The emphasis on collective responsibility leads to the belief that mental illness is a family problem. Care-giving is thus retained within the context of the family for as long as possible, which results in delay in getting professional help (Ryder, Bean, & Dion, 2000). About 80% of Japanese respondents agreed with a landlord's decision not to rent a house to someone with mental illness (Tanaka, Inadomi, Kikuchi, & Ohta, 2006). The foregoing demonstrates that the form and nature may differ across cultures, but stigmatisation of mental illness is present in all societies and all classes of people.

Demographic Correlates of Stigmatising Attitudes

Research indicates that particular groups in society are more likely than others to display negative attitudes. Education, age, familiarity with persons with mental illness, gender, religious affiliation, and profession predict attitudes towards people with mental illness to varying degrees (Angermeyer & Dietrich, 2006; Ikwuka, 2016). Papadopoulos and colleagues (2002) observed that the most consistent predictor of stigma was knowledge level, with higher knowledge scores correlating with decreased stigma. The case study of south-eastern Nigeria (Ikwuka, 2016) replicated the findings of Arvaniti and colleagues (2009) that people with more education supported social integration of persons with mental illness, were less discriminatory and less supportive of socially restricting them, while less education predicted most of the negative attitudes including authoritarian treatment, social restrictions, and keeping a distance from them both at primary and secondary levels of association. This agrees with a study of Northern Nigeria which found that literate respondents were seven times more likely to demonstrate positive attitudes towards people with mental illness compared to illiterate respondents (Kabir, Iliyasu, Abubakar, & Aliyu, 2004). They were equally less moralistic and judgmental and had greater treatment optimism (Richmond & Foster, 2003).

Ikwuka (2016) also found that older age was associated with more social restrictive, less pro-community care, and less benevolent attitudes towards people with mental illness. It was also associated with more desire for social distance at secondary levels of association. These findings agree with studies that identify the old with generally more negative attitudes (Papadopoulos, Leavey, & Vincent, 2002; Riedel-Heller, Matschinger & Angermeyer, 2005; Shulman & Adams, 2002). As the custodians of tradition, the old are associated with more pre-scientific and supernatural causal views which have been linked with negative attitudes towards mental illness (Adewuya & Makanjuola, 2008; Gureje, Olley, Ephraim-Oluwanuga, & Kola, 2006; Song, Chang, Shih, Lin, & Yang, 2005). Furthermore, in their perceived concern for social equilibrium (Stuart & Arbodela-Flórez, 2001a), the old would be more averse to situations they consider to be potentially disruptive.

However, Ikwuka (2016) reported that the young demonstrated a more authoritarian attitude than the old, which agrees with the observation that the young are more fearful of violence and more likely to associate mental illness with it (Crisp et al., 2000; Pinfold et al., 2003). Kobau and colleagues (2010) also found that young adults aged 18–24 years were more inclined towards negative stereotypes, and were also more pessimistic about treatment and prognosis, which might dissuade them from seeking treatment in times of need. Stigma is under-researched in adolescents, covering less than 4% of stigma research (Link, Yang, Phelan, & Collins, 2004), yet this group was found to be less likely to receive appropriate care (Department of Health and Human Services, 1999). Stigma reduction during the adolescent years is important for early detection and early treatment and increasing adolescents' comfort in discussing mental disorders (Pinto-Foltz & Logsdon, 2009). The foregoing suggests that when broken down, some aspects of stigmatising attitudes may be more pronounced within particular groups (Hannigan, 1999). Hence anti-stigma campaigns might be more effective with targeted than general interventions.

The case study of south-eastern Nigeria equally found that males endorsed more social restriction of people with mental illness, were less supportive of caring for them in the community and their social integration than females. This agrees with many research findings indicating that males demonstrate more negative attitudes towards mental illness than females (Kobau, DiIorio, Chapman & Delvecchio, 2010; Marie & Miles, 2008). Male negative attitudes could result from traditional masculine social roles which disapproved of expressiveness in illness behaviour (Addis & Mahalik, 2003; Moller-Leimkuhler, 2002). Males are equally far less knowledgeable about health in general (Courtenay, 2000) and mental health, in particular (Cotton, Wright, Harris, Jorm, & McGorry, 2006).

On the other hand, gender differences within relationships could provide an insight into why females demonstrate more positive attitudes towards people with mental illness. Maccoby (1990) suggests that females' social interaction patterns are of the 'enabling style' that fosters greater equality and intimacy and keeps the interaction continuing whereas males tend to exhibit the 'constructing style' to inhibit their partners or cause the partner to withdraw, shorten the interaction, or bring it to an end. Consequently, females were found to be more willing to foster social interaction with persons with mental illness and support their integration in schools and the community (Antonak & Harth, 1994; Gash & Coffey, 1995).

However, Dessoki and Hifnawy (2009) suggest that females tend to be more negative towards mental illness in cultures that discriminate against women. In these cultures, women may be the greater sufferers from the stigma of mental illness with regard to reduced marital opportunities and the increased risk of divorce in an existing marriage, should the condition become public. Supporting this notion is the finding that a higher number of men receive hospital treatment for schizophrenia in Morocco which suggests that stigma is greater for women, as few women come forward for treatment (Kadri, Manoudi, Berrada, & Moussaoui, 2004).

Controversy remains over how and to what extent religiosity and denominational affiliation influence attitudes and behaviour on social issues.

Religious affiliation is however associated with conservatism in some aspects of socio-ethical worldviews, with Evangelical Protestants and Catholics, for instance, being more pro-family and pro-life than mainstream Protestants (Waldman, 2019). This seems a plausible ideological background to the finding in the case study of south-eastern Nigeria that Protestants desired social distance from people with mental illness significantly more than the Catholics at both primary and secondary levels of association. Catholic beliefs are based on a strong principle of the right to life (Jelen, 1984), and therefore less subject to the challenges of extenuating circumstances, including disability. Furthermore, an earlier study of south-eastern Nigeria (Ikwuka, Nyatanga & Galbraith, 2014) found that compared to the Catholics, mainstream Protestants were more supernatural in their causal attribution for mental illness, which is associated with more negative attitudes. It is suggested that the more independent Protestant denomination tends to be more indigenised than the West-mediated "Roman" Catholic Church (Meyer, 2004). The findings heighten the prospect of collaborating with religious leaders to improve notions of mental illness and reduce stigma through targeting of religious misattributions about the aetiology and dangerousness of mental illness.

More than half of the nurses surveyed in the case study of south-eastern Nigeria endorsed authoritarian attitudes towards people with mental illness and maintenance of social distance from them at primary levels of association. This is comparable to the findings with the non-nursing groups (students, teachers, and the general public). It is a disturbing finding given that nurses are major providers of hospital care. Studies have noted the adverse impact of negative attitudes in the provision of care (Sharrock & Happell, 2002), (see also Chapter 8, Experience of the Mental Health System). In one study, nurses were less optimistic about treatment outcomes of mental illness than the public (Hugo, 2001).

Clinical observation bias has been cited as one reason why professionals, especially nurses, develop negative attitudes towards persons with mental illness (Grausgruber, Meise, Katschnig, Schöny, & Fleischhacker, 2007; Hugo, 2001). This suggests that staff in in-patient clinical services often see chronic patients with poorer prognosis while people with better outcomes present more as out-patients, away from the regular view of staff working in more intensive settings. Constant exposure to, and encounter with, chronic patients could, therefore lead to therapeutic pessimism and a biased view of the client's potential. This agrees with Bailey (1998) who found a predominantly negative experience of nurses' care for psychiatric patients in general wards owing to lack of positive feedback. Negative attitudes may also stem from negative professional experiences with patients with chronic mental illness, especially from those suffering from paranoid schizophrenia, who could display aggressive behaviour that could lead to distancing behaviour from health workers.

Among health workers, nurses have been noted as being most prone to suffer violence at the hands of patients (Cooper & Swanson, 2002; Whittington & Higgins, 2002). However, generally, negative professional attitudes stem from a lack of knowledge, frustration, and a sense of inadequacy in handling the difficulties posed by this client group (Gafoor & Rassool, 1998; Thomas, 1995). Studies highlight the importance of training programmes to improve the practical and theoretical knowledge of nurses (Lowe, Bond, Spokes, & Wellman, 2002; Needham, Abderhalden, Dassen, Haug, & Fischer, 2002). These were found to improve confidence and increase treatment optimism (McConachie & Whitford, 2009; Gerace, Hughes, & Spunt, 1995).

General nurses, studied by Reed and Fitzgerald (2005), who disliked and avoided caring for patients with mental illness because they felt inadequate, displayed positive attitudes when given support. The benefit of the experience of these nurses could explain the promising finding in the case study (ikwuka, 2016) where they displayed significantly more pro-community care attitude, and less of all the negative attitudes, compared to the non-nursing groups. This agrees with an earlier study (Olade, 1979) that compared the attitudes of post-basic nursing students with those of science students in south-western Nigeria. The nursing students demonstrated more favourable attitudes towards mental illness, scoring higher in Interpersonal Aetiology and Mental Hygiene, and lower in Authoritarianism and Social Restrictiveness. Since nurses could be responding more positively to agree with the expectations of their profession, comparing the attitudes of general nurses with those of psychiatric nurses could help to substantiate the merits of training on mental health and the contact theory (see Chapter 6) for attitude improvement.

Teachers in the case study not only replicated the general public's pattern of negative attitudes across the attitude constructs but were actually less pro-community care. This reflects the finding of another Nigerian survey (Aghukwa, 2009b) whereby four in five teachers felt that psychiatric inpatients should be surrounded by high walls and guards. This suggests that teachers are no better than the parents and their school-going children in their understanding of mental illness. It is a disturbing finding given the critical role of teachers in the attitude formation of pupils, including some who may be experiencing mental illness. It demonstrates that in the war against stigma, merely being educated, which does not easily eradicate culturally enshrined beliefs, (Adewuya & Oguntade, 2007; Ikwuka, Galbraith, & Nyatanga, 2014) is not enough. There is a specific need for mental health education that addresses mental illness stigma.

In the case study of south-eastern Nigeria, the UK-based respondents displayed significantly less negative attitudes compared with the home-(Nigeria) based group with regard to the desire for social distance both at the primary and the secondary levels of association. It is to be expected that social conditioning (acculturation) could be a factor here whereby the experience of the host (UK) culture, with a more developed and open healthcare system, as well as mental health charities and campaigns for the rights of persons with mental illness, would have influenced the attitudes of the UK-based respondents. Corroborating this, a study observed that shorter residence in the United States was associated with more negative attitudes toward mental health services (Jang, Kim, Hansen, & Chiriboga, 2007).

Yet, that almost two-thirds (63.6%) and 41.2% of the UK-based sample still endorsed social distance at the primary and secondary levels of association, respectively, is a cause for concern. It indicates the disturbing possibility that this immigrant population could relate to persons experiencing mental illness with prejudice in a culture that is less accepting of such discriminatory attitudes. This could fuel conflict. Moreover, the finding could have implications for their own mental healthcare as immigrants in a Western host culture. For instance, it could lead to self-stigmatisation by someone suffering from mental illness and stigmatisation of psychiatric services. These, in turn, could lead to poor help-seeking behaviour. Secondly, when it leads to lowered self-esteem, it could further impact negatively on adjustment, which might already be potentially threatened by their migrant status. The finding thus underscores the limitations of social conditioning in moderating culturally held beliefs. The improvement of attitudes towards mental illness and sufferers cannot, therefore, be left to the dynamics of acculturation and social change. There is a need for a formal system of engaging immigrant groups towards improving notions of mental illness.

A UK study (Wolff, Pathare, Craig, & Leff, 1996) noted that minority ethnic groups were more likely to hold negative attitudes towards mental illness than white British-born. Explaining the difference, the authors suggested that minority ethnic respondents were more likely than the white UK-born group to object to an educational campaign. Yet, insights from causal mechanisms studies highlight the significance of variables such as language barrier (Maughan, 2005), socio-economic constraints (Walters, 2001), the atmosphere of mutual mistrust between the system and the ethnic minorities (Gillborn & Gibbs, 1996) (see also Chapter 7, Cultural (In)appropriateness of Care) and, as the foregoing suggests, the carried-over cultural background of the immigrants in mediating such disparities.

Since attitude change does not necessarily translate to behaviour change (Krauss, 1995), factors such as individual differences in stigmatising attitudes and responding to stigma-reduction strategies need to be explored. Targeted campaigns to stem mental illness stigma have proved much more successful than mounting massive general public efforts as one size does not fit all (Arboleda-Flórez, 2001) hence the importance of determining the demographic correlates of stigmatising attitudes.

6 Improving Stigmatising Attitudes

Very few studies report on practical methods that can be adopted to combat stigmatised attitudes (Rao et al., 2009). However, based on a review of the literature from social psychology, three approaches to addressing public stigma have emerged: education, contact and advocacy (Corrigan, Druss, & Perlick, 2014). The World Psychiatric Association utilises these three approaches (Satorius, 1997). Education replaces stigma with accurate conceptions about the disorders. Promotion of contact challenges public attitudes about mental illness through direct interactions with persons who have these disorders. Advocacy seeks to suppress stigmatising attitudes to mental illness and behaviours that promote these attitudes. However, the results of these interventions have been generally modest, and even contradictory, suggesting the complexity of attitude change.

Education

The central role of education in improving attitudes was immediately evident in the case study of south-eastern Nigeria (Ikwuka, 2016) where a low level of education associated significantly more with all the negative attitude constructs compared with a higher level of education which was associated significantly more with the positive attitude constructs. The importance of education in shaping attitudes was such that levels of education were found to be associated with levels of attitudinal dispositions in a study: respondents with postgraduate qualifications held less negative attitudes towards persons with mental illness than those with a first degree; those with a first degree, in turn, were less stigmatising than those with lower qualifications in respect of responsibility, anger, dangerousness, fear and social distance (Aghukwa, 2010).

However, studies demonstrate that, beyond being formally educated, positive attitudes are enhanced more specifically with mental health education which disconfirms stereotypes with accurate conceptions and evidence-based insights (Corrigan & Penn, 1999; Corrigan et al., 2014; Gureje, Olley, Ephraim-Oluwanuga, & Kola, 2006). Mental health literacy encompasses knowledge about preventing disorders, recognising them when they develop, pursuing help when disorders become distressing, and using mental health first aid skills to support others in distress (Corrigan et al., 2014). Enlightenment campaigns that address minority-group stereotypes have used books, videos, slides, and other audiovisual aids to highlight false assumptions about groups and provide facts that counter these assumptions. When augmented by discussions, such didactic formats lead to participants' rejection of false assumptions and recalling of accurate information (Corrigan & Penn, 1999).

Trained psychiatric nurses and doctors expressed more positive feelings towards mental illness than non-psychiatric trained registered nurses in south-western Nigeria (Odejide & Olatawura, 1979). Similarly, while a study that examined the attitudes of primary health workers without prior exposure to mental health training in the region revealed that 72% of them expressed negative attitudes towards patients of mental illness (Abiodun, 1991), a later educational intervention with rural community mental health volunteers in the region led to a significant reduction in the perceived dangerousness of people with mental illness and a significant reduction in the degree of the social distance they desired from them (Abayomi, Adelufosi, & Olajide, 2013).

Moreover, in an earlier appraisal of an interventionist programme using the Opinion about Mental Illness (OMI) Scale (Olade, 1983), a two-year assessment of the effect of integrating mental health concepts into a post-basic nursing degree programme was carried out with two classes of students with minimal psychiatric preparation in their diploma programme. They were studied as they progressed from first to second year, and from second to third year, at the three-year post-basic nursing degree programme at the University of Ibadan, south-western Nigeria. Results showed changes in both groups in terms of amelioration of both authoritarian and socially restrictive attitudes. Similarly, there were significant changes in knowledge and beliefs about mental illness following a four-week psychiatric rotation, on the beliefs and attitudes of final-year medical students from a north-western Nigerian University (Aghukwa, 2010).

When a one-hour educational programme, developed to change attitudes towards mental illness, was introduced for medical students to investigate its effects on their attitudes, more students indicated a willingness to accept former patients at relatively closer proximity after the programme (Mino, Yasuda, Tsuda, & Shimodera, 2001). Favourable attitudinal changes were observed in terms of psychiatric services, the human rights of persons with mental illness, patients' independence in social life, and the causes and characteristics of mental illness. Significantly more students respected the rights of persons with mental illness to divorce their spouses, and their right to vote. Similarly, four out of five OMI factors changed in a favourable, and statistically significant direction following mental health course work: Authoritarianism, Mental Hygiene Ideology, Social Restrictiveness and Interpersonal Aetiology. Only Unsophisticated Benevolence did not show a significant change (Neil, Penny & MS OTR/L, 2002).

Medical students who had completed their course in psychiatry demonstrated more positive attitudes towards the social integration of patients than pre-clinical medical students, who held attitudes similar to those of the general population (Ay, Save, & Fidanoglu, 2006; Mukherjee, Fialho, Wijetunge, Chesinski, & Surgenor, 2002). A study in the United Kingdom found less mental health stigma among doctors compared with medical students and members of the public in that order (Mukherjee et al., 2002).

Through the provision of information and increased opportunity to gain more scientific knowledge about characteristics of illnesses, including causation, prevention and the possibility of effective treatments, mental health education challenges certain negative traditional beliefs. It introduces some evidence-based biomedical and psychosocial alternatives, enlightens the public to make more informed decisions about mental illness, challenges people with stigmatising attitudes to reflect on their feelings and leads to some form of circumspection (Haghighat, 2001; Monteith, 1996; Mulatu, 1999). Consequently, mental health education demonstrates that:

1   Mental illness is indeed like any other illness as most people with mental illness retain many of their capacities (Sartorius, 2002). Some people with serious mental illness like schizophrenia have demonstrated the ability to live with recurring auditory hallucinations without distress, pursue a career, and enjoy a full family life (Ralph & Corrigan, 2005).

2   Mental disorders can be effectively treated or managed (WHO, 2001a; Kobau, DiIorio, Chapman, & Delvecchio, 2010).

3   The public grossly overestimates the dangerousness and violence of people with mental illness (Swanson et al., 2002, 2006), and often inaccurately ascribes particularly heinous crimes, such as mass shootings, to mental illness (Corrigan & Watson, 2005).

4   Violence is not necessarily an essential attribute of psychoses, as the potential for violence is oftentimes heightened by intervening co-morbid factors such as alcohol and drug abuse, treatment non-compliance, lack of knowledge about the condition, poverty, homelessness and a history of violence and criminality (Aghukwa, 2009a; Department of Health, 2001; Soyka, 2000).

5   Not all serious mental illnesses lead to obvious or disruptive behaviour. For instance, patients with schizophrenia can have predominantly negative symptoms (Sadock & Sadock, 2007).

6   Mental disorders account for less violence in society than do alcohol and drug abuse (Brunton, 1997; Eronen, Tihonen, & Hakola, 1996).
7   People with mental illness are actually more likely to be the victims rather than the perpetrators of violence (Department of Health, 2003). Vagrants suffering from psychosis ('mad people') in Nigeria experience repeated verbal, physical and sexual abuses (Adesomoju, 2013; Aghukwa, 2009a). They are exploited for money-making, used in circus shows and for rituals with some dying at the hands of society.

Well-resourced educational programmes should aim at helping people develop a strong sense of understanding, empathy, compassion, and tolerance towards persons with mental illness and survivors. Such programmes should help people understand that persons with mental illness are not essentially different from people with such chronic physical health conditions as diabetes, hypertension, or heart diseases. The public should be made to understand that with advances in the treatment of mental health problems and community support, many survivors of mental illness could live fulfilled lives and contribute to the progress of their community.

Mental health education has been linked with shifts from superstitious beliefs to modern biomedical beliefs and practices in Ethiopia, as well as in other sub-Saharan African countries (Mulatu, 1999). By providing increased opportunities to gain more scientific knowledge about characteristics of illnesses, including causation and prevention, education may also lessen the negative attitudes directed towards patients. Carrying out enlightenment campaigns, beginning with groups at most risk of displaying negative attitudes (as highlighted in the preceding chapter 5) will be very pertinent. Mental health education and enlightenment should also start from an early age as attitudes are formed during childhood and once formed, can be hard to change (Putman, 2009). It makes sense to support the development of positive attitudes from an early age when there is cognitive flexibility rather than to struggle to change them in adulthood.

Contact

While existing literature has consistently found that better knowledge of mental illness is associated with reduced stigmatising attitudes, in a study of south-eastern Nigeria (Uwakwe, 2007), medical students did not differ in their beliefs even after their four weeks of schedule in mental health. Non-mental health workers in a study of north-eastern Nigeria, who demonstrated a good understanding of the biopsychosocial cause of mental illness still exhibited prominent negative attitudes (Oderinde et al. 2018). In a study of the British populace, Byrne (1997) found that, despite more than half of the study sample having had a fair knowledge of mental illness, the majority held negative attitudes towards persons with mental illness. Similarly, population surveys in Germany showed an increase in mental health literacy but no change in the desire for social distance (Angermeyer, Holzinger, & Matschinger, 2009).

Many studies have also failed to find a direct relationship between stigmatising opinions and lack of knowledge of mental illness even among mental health service providers (Crisp, Gelder, Rix, Meltzer, & Rowlands, 2000; Kingdon, Sharma, & Hart, 2004; Mukherjee et al., 2002). An earlier study from Turkey even found higher levels of negative attitude among health workers with higher education than those with less education (Aydin, Yigit, Inandi, & Kirpinar, 2003). Against this background, the consistent research finding that attitudes improve the most when theoretical knowledge is complemented with experiential knowledge, that is, with contact with persons with mental illnesses (Angermeyer, Matschinger, & Corrigan, 2004; Bjo¨rkman, Angelman, & Jönsson, 2008; Corrigan & O'Shaughnessy, 2007; Rusch, Angermeyer, & Corrigan, 2005) becomes compelling.

Indeed, research suggests that theoretical knowledge without contact could increase social distance (Chou & Mak, 1998). As observed with education, the scale of contact is positively associated with an improvement of attitude. This was evident among physicians, whereby General Practitioners with over ten years of experience demonstrated more favourable and more lucid views of patients with mental illness than House Officers (Khoweiled, 2005). Afana and colleagues (2000) equally showed in their study, which explored the attitudes of 166 Palestinian primary health care professionals, that older professionals demonstrated more empathetic and tolerant attitudes. Ndetei and colleagues (2012) found that older nurses and older doctors in the profession had less stigmatising attitudes which may have risen from more clinical exposure and awareness in the course of their practice and experience.

In Nigeria, where it is not unusual to see children taunt persons with mental illness (a behaviour that continues well into adulthood), a study that determined the effect of a three-day mental health training programme for school pupils, on the perceptions of, and social distance towards persons with mental illness in the south-western region showed that multiple contacts and mixed-method training sessions produced a positive and sustained change in knowledge of, and attitude towards, persons with mental illness (Adeola, Babatunde, & Olayinka, 2017). Desforges and colleagues (1991) carefully examined the effects of strategic contact in a laboratory study with 95 undergraduates in a randomised controlled trial. After participating in a cooperative task with a person described as recently released from a mental institution, students, who were initially prejudiced, endorsed more positive attitudes about the person with mental illness and showed greater acceptance toward mental illness in general.

Education has been found to reduce stereotyping views but not social distancing (Dietrich, Heider, Matschinger, & Angermeyer, 2006). Going by the theory of social representations, the notion of the 'stigma process' (Link, Struening, Rahav, Phelan, & Nuttbrock, 1997) seems particularly suitable for explaining this phenomenon. According to this model, the various stigma components can be conceived of as being arranged in a logical order with stereotyping coming first and discrimination (the desire for social distance) following. The exposure to educational (enlightenment) materials may first affect the stereotypes held by people (i.e. the cognitive stigma component), before the desire for social distance (i.e. their behavioural intentions) will also be changed. Indeed, Schulze and colleagues (2003) found that it is easier to change stereotypes than behavioural intentions. However, though attitude change does not necessarily translate to behaviour change, the association is strengthened if attitudes are accessible, stable, formed as a result of direct experience, and personally relevant (Krauss, 1995; Petty, 1995).

Research has demonstrated that members of the majority group who have met persons representing a minority group are more likely to disconfirm stereotypes describing that group (Gaertner, Rust, Dovidio, Bachman, & Anastasio, 1996). Experimental studies indicate that among the available strategies: education, advocacy and contact with persons with mental illness, the latter may be the most effective in inducing change (Corrigan et al., 2002). A meta-analysis showed contact with someone with mental illness yielding significantly better effects than education on attitudes about and behaviour intentions towards people with mental illness (Corrigan, Morris, Michaels, Rafacz, & Rüsch, 2012).

Both personal and professional contacts with people with mental illness have been linked to reduced stigma. Findings indicate that people with more experiential information about mental illness such as relatives of people with schizophrenia are less prejudicial, less critical, more tolerant and desire less social distance from people with mental illness (Alexander & Link, 2003; Angermeyer et al., 2004; Hannigan, 1999; Högberg, Magnusson, Ewertzon, & Lützén, 2008). A large-scale survey of approximately 5,000 US adults revealed that those who knew someone with a mental illness or who had ever had a mental illness themselves were less inclined to have negative stereotypes and had more positive views regarding prognosis following treatment (Kobau et al., 2010). Huxley (1993) found that respondents who were less embarrassed by mental illness were more likely to know someone who is receiving help and treatment at the community facility. In a conservative, more superstitious, morally, and socially judgmental south-western Nigerian society, Odejide and Olatawura (1979) claimed that the effect of the day-to-day interaction of the psychiatric nurses with persons with mental illness so improved their attitude towards them that many of the psychiatric nursing respondents held no objection to marrying ex-psychiatric patients.

Conversely, lack of experiential knowledge (either through personal experience or closeness to others who had experienced or were experiencing mental illness) was associated with more negative attitudes including the desire for social distance and social control (Brockington, Hall, Levings, & Murray, 1993). This is corroborated by the case study of south-eastern Nigeria (Ikwuka, 2016) whereby those not familiar with someone or persons with mental illness significantly endorsed more authoritarian attitudes and desired more social distance from such people than those familiar with them.

Contact entails strategic interactions between people with lived experience of mental illness and targeted members of the public (Couture & Penn, 2003). The interaction mediated by contact disconfirms the stereotype held by those without mental disorders. Contact theory proposes that contact decreases negative attitudes through cognitive individuation especially when the contact is auspicious – personal, intensive, extensive, equal, voluntary, and within a meaningful, supportive context (Corrigan & Penn, 1999; Penny, Kasar, & Sinay, 2000; Wallach, 2004; Weller & Grunes 1988).

Arboleda-Flórez (2001) observes that some successful strategies in combating stigma usually include the participation of care providers and the patients or consumers themselves. The strategies that have worked include those that train and organise individual consumers, or patients, and their families to provide talks to such specialised groups as students, nurses, or businesspeople, about their mental illness and how they are coping and managing their lives. Very effective in this regard is dramatised illustration by consumers themselves of the distress of patients and the additional impact of stigma and discrimination. Making the public 'experience' the suffering of persons with mental illness can make them more sympathetic, considerate, and possibly less stigmatising. Thus, members of the disability community had developed simulations of mental illness to help persons who are not disabled understand their plight (Kiger, 1992). In one of such exercises, participants experience the intrusive nature of auditory hallucinations by trying to complete simple work tasks while listening to an audiotape of irrelevant and mixed-up voices.

Consistent with the social learning theory, researchers suggest that teaching agents who are relatively similar to the pupil are likely to have the most impact, hence peers can be especially potent teachers (Calhoun et al., 2010). Thus, regular involvement of mental health service users in teaching sessions where possible is a positive way of reducing negative attitudes and of improving understanding of mental illness (Putman, 2008). Targeting the associative stigma of the mental health profession, an education programme delivered by a psychiatrist to high school students on mental health issues was found to increase both the appreciation of practitioners and care-seeking (Battaglia, Coverdale, & Bushong, 1990). Real-life interaction is more rewarding than virtual or arranged meetings (Sigelman & Welch, 1993). Attitudes based on direct experience have been found to be more influential in predicting later behaviour than those based on learning material (Fazio, 1990).

However, contact should be with a representative member of the population, such as someone who may still grapple with residual symptoms but who is fairly well integrated, for instance, capable of independent living, rather than with an exceptional member of the population like someone whose symptoms are completely remitted (Angermeyer & Matschinger, 1997; Corrigan & Penn, 1999; Desforges et al., 1991). Contact with an 'atypical' member may be sub-typed as unusual, and sub-typing insulates the broader stereotype (Kunda & Oleson, 1995, 1997). Thus, the nature of the contact is a critical factor in the workability of contact theory. Brief exposure can be detrimental and could increase social restrictiveness (Wallach, 2004). Keane (1991) suggested that brief contact with people with chronic severe mental illness contributes to a sense of hopelessness in students.

As Kermode and colleagues (2009) observed, perception of dangerousness may be more difficult to address if it is generated by personal experience with people who are in a crisis with their condition. This agrees with Corrigan and colleague's (2005) submission that contact can worsen a stereotype if the type of person interacted with reinforces it. Some negative experiences such as a difficult or distant family relationship, a troubled marriage to a person with mental illness, a threatening public encounter with a stranger who appears to suffer from mental illness or negative experiences in the workplace would likely have no positive impact or have a negative one upon stigmatising attitudes (Alexander & Link, 2003). However, education can help in clarifying peculiar situations and possible intervening co-morbid risk factors. Such a combination of education and face-to-face interaction (experience) as is presently done in campaigns against stigma towards people living with HIVAIDS (Brown, Trujillo, & Macintyre, 2001) could have a greater impact on changing attitudes towards people with mental illness than using either strategy in isolation.

Advocacy

Development of national policies and legislation has the potential for the most impact in a stigma reduction effort (Addison & Thorpe, 2004; Crisp et al., 2000; Department of Health, 2003). Such paths have been successfully taken in the campaigns for racial equality and rights for the physically disabled (Disability Discrimination Act, 2005). The effectiveness of organised awareness activities in combating the stigma of mental illness has been recognised and includes initiatives such as World Mental Health Day (October 10 each year) and Mental Health Awareness Week. It also includes becoming a "stigma-buster" (by recognising and being ready to denounce news, advertisements, or movies that stigmatise, ridicule, demonise, misrepresent, or stereotype people with mental illness as violent, unpredictable, or dangerous) or to be part of a pressure group that highlights the sufferings persons with mental illness face in securing proper housing and employment, and in accessing treatment or using public facilities.

Another effective way to raise awareness is the facilitation of consumer movements (involving consumers and their families) from local groups to national alliances for mental health that would collaborate with national professional bodies such as the National Psychiatric, Psychological, Nurses, or Social Workers' Associations. These bodies can speak with authority to national governments on behalf of persons with mental illness and could be stimulated to lobby the government to introduce legislation that combats stigma and that outlaws discrimination, whether based on group characteristics or individual physical or mental disabilities.

Arboleda-Flórez (2001) chronicled the following national and international efforts to help combat stigma, underscoring the decisive interventions of such bodies as the World Health Organisation (WHO) and the World Psychiatric Association (WPA) in the welfare of people with mental illness. In 1996, the World Psychiatric Association began an initiative – the *Open the Doors* programme, to combat the stigma associated with schizophrenia and increase mental health knowledge. *Open the Doors* is collaborative, multi-centred, and involves family and patient organisations. It encourages action to decrease prejudice and discrimination. Outreach is driven from the perspective of those experiencing stigma as opposed to established mental health theories that may not have been tested in diverse cultures (Okasha, 2007).

Open the Doors recognises cultural, socio-economic, and demographic differences. It targets different demographics according to locations but depends heavily on local action groups which organise themselves to plan and initiate projects that mobilise local resources into action to combat the stigma associated with the mental illness in question. The programme produced five volumes containing how-to guidelines and information on schizophrenia. The first volume is a step-by-step how-to guide to develop local programmes. The second volume is a compendium of the latest knowledge on the diagnosis and treatment of schizophrenia, including psychosocial reintegration strategies. The third includes reports from a number of countries while the fourth is a collection of reports from other countries where similar initiatives are on-going or being planned. The final volume contains an annotated bibliography of practical materials which can all be downloaded from the WPA Programme website.

The WPA has used psycho-educational interventions to combat stigma and discrimination related to mental illness in more than 20 countries (Pinfold, Stuart, Thornicroft, & Arboleda-Florez, 2005). It begins with an examination of experiences that patients and their families have had since the onset of the illness, which serves to select targets for interventions that will aim to reduce stigma and its consequences. It involves different social sectors such as health ministries, social welfare services, labour ministries, non-governmental organisations, and the media. It is a long-term engagement with a different focus for different settings. One of the first targets of the programme in Canada was a change in procedures used in emergency departments that discriminated against people with mental illness. The attitudes of the shopkeepers were the target in Italy while the media was the focus in Germany. The procedure highlighted certain themes as well as sources of stigmatisation often neglected, namely, the behaviour of medical professionals, particularly the psychiatrists.

The World Health Organisation (2001c) launched its initiative *Stop Exclusion, Dare to Care* which aimed at combating stigma and rallying support for more enlightened and equitable structures for dealing with mental illness, and the acceptance of mental health as a major topic of concern among member states. The initiative was conceptualised to follow cognitive methodologies for behavioural change. The three major goals were: to increase awareness and knowledge of the nature of mental illness, to improve public attitudes toward those who suffer from mental illness and their families, and to generate action to prevent and eliminate stigma and discrimination.

The programme called on individuals, families, communities, the media, NGOs, professionals, scientists, policymakers etc. to join forces and to share a vision where individuals recognise the importance of their own mental health, and sufferers, families and communities feel sufficiently empowered to address their own mental health needs. Professionals will treat, as well as engage actively in mental health promotion and preventative activities, and policymakers will draw up policies that are more responsive to the needs of the entire population. The programme makes a wake-up call on the global scale of mental illness with about 45 million persons worldwide suffering from schizophrenia alone, and it illustrates how the majority of these persons are deprived of even the most basic treatments. The programme underscores the need for mental health to be incorporated into the general healthcare services of countries. It underlines the ethical responsibility of nations to be inclusive of all citizens and respect their human rights. It also aims at providing incentives to governments and healthcare bodies to review policies and to become actively involved in the reorganisation of services and the development of responsive mental health policies.

For more than a hundred years, the National Mental Health Association (Mental Health America, MHA), has been engaged in the mission of promoting mental health and preventing mental illness through advocacy, education, research, and services. The organisation collaborates with a wide audience of over 200 affiliates and supporters to advance policy recommendations that promote improved attitudes toward mental illness, improved services for people with mental illness, prevention of mental illnesses and the promotion of overall mental health of all.

MHA is driven by a commitment to promote mental health as a critical part of overall wellness, including prevention services for all, early identification, and intervention for those at risk, integrated care, services, and supports for those who need them, with recovery as the goal. It works to protect the rights and dignity of individuals who live with mental illness nationwide and ensures that their voices are integrated into all areas of the organisation with a focus on inclusion, self-directed care, and recovery. The body helps citizens of all ages better understand prevention, early identification, and intervention through a variety of information, online tools, and events. In their anti-stigma campaigns, they also constructively engage the popular mainstream media, which are key culprits in the dissemination of messages that stigmatise persons with mental illness. They sponsor films and television shows that disseminate stigma-countering information.

Similarly, the National Alliance on Mental Illness (NAMI), America's largest grassroots mental health organisation, works to eliminate the stigma associated with mental disorders and improve the quality of life for sufferers. NAMI started as a small group of concerned families but has risen to an association of more than 500 local affiliates that work in communities to raise awareness and provide support and education that was not previously available to those in need. NAMI uses stigma-busters, protest, personal contact, and community education. Stigma-busters approach media people who inaccurately portray mental disorders and demand that they stop inaccurate portrayal. Corrigan and Penn (1999) reported that NAMI worked with CBS to produce the Marie Balter Story, a movie about the struggle and successes of a woman who had been institutionalised for more than a decade. CBS and Hallmark Cards aired the film *Promise* in which James Woods and James Gamer depicted the real-life interactions of a man with schizophrenia and his brother. Media efforts are influential because of their wide reach.

In Our Own Voice, a manualised contact and educational programme of NAMI is designed to increase mental health knowledge and reduce stigma. It consists of two consumers (people who have recovered from a mental disorder and have received *In Our Own Voice* training) sharing their experiences of living with, and recovering from, a mental disorder. *In Our Own Voice* has been presented to lay and professional audiences. NAMI also passed out "media watch kits" to local affiliates for monitoring newspapers, television, and periodicals in their area.

Corrigan and Penn (1999) also reported that Paramount Pictures changed marketing strategies for patently offensive newspaper and poster ads for a film titled "Crazy People" with a picture of a cracked egg with hands and arms and the caption "Warning: Crazy people are coming", after a discussion with representatives from several advocacy groups. A new ad that had pictures of the film's stars Dudley Moore and Daryl Hannah, with the revised header, "You wanna laugh tonight?" was used instead. As a Philadelphia newspaper was promoting the movie by offering free admission to persons who could prove they were "crazy", the local advocacy groups wrote letters, marched outside newspaper offices, and met with the newspaper's publisher until the marketing scheme was stopped. Examples like these suggest that protest reduces the frequency of publicly endorsed stereotypes.

The U.S. Department of Health and Human Services Substance Abuse and Mental Health Service Administration (SAMHSA) publishes a quarterly memorandum that reports advances in stigma research and highlights successful stigma-reduction programmes. SAMHSA hosts teleconference training approximately six times a year to advance knowledge about stigma and stigma reduction and to foster partnerships between consumer groups, businesses, local government agencies, and other organisations interested in combating stigma. SAMHSA also offers a free resource tool kit *Developing a Stigma Reduction Initiative* to raise awareness about mental health and assist organisations in fighting stigma.

The Royal College of Psychiatrists in the UK organised the five-year *Changing Mind* campaign aimed at dispelling myths and stereotypes about mental illness and sufferers by challenging misrepresentations and discrimination, encouraging patient advocacy and educating the public on the real nature and treatability of mental disorders (Crisp et al., 2000). The campaign used leaflets, pamphlets, films and other mass communication facilities. In one well-known film, "1 in 4", the message is direct and pithy as it emphasises that mental health problems can touch anyone. The film proclaims that one in four could be your Brother, your Sister, your Wife, your Girlfriend, your Daughter; one in four could be me, it could be you. The UK's *Time to Change* initiative also seeks to promote care and to challenge discrimination so that people with mental illness will have opportunities that are similar to those of everyone else. Awareness of *Time to Change* ranged between 38% and 64% and was associated with greater mental health literacy and less stigmatising attitudes (Evans-Lacko, Corker, Williams, Henderson, & Thornicraft, 2014).

With the aim of improving mental health literacy in the population, the Australia Department of Health and Aged Care (1998) facilitated campaigns such as the Australian National Community Awareness Program (CAP). The three goals of CAP include: to position mental health on the public agenda, to promote a greater understanding and acceptance of those with mental illness, and to dispel myths and misconceptions about mental illness. Though tolerant attitudes were not found to increase following the programme, they were consolidated, and there was a slight increase in the awareness of services. Furthermore, prompted by service users and carers' concerns about the stigmatising attitudes of health professionals in Australia, one objective of the National Mental Health Policy was to address the attitudes of mental health professionals (Hugo, 2001). The Australasian Psychiatric Stigma Group links consumers, providers, and other interest groups, in a public evaluation of the impact of stereotyping and stigma on the lives of psychiatric service-users, their carers, and the lives of providers (Rosen, Walter, Casey, & Hocking, 2000).

Following a nationally representative survey of the Australian population (Jorm, Korten, Jacomb, Christensen, & Pollitt, 1997) which found that the public had poor mental health literacy that could impede early detection and appropriate help-seeking behaviour, the authors designed mental health first-aid training courses for the general public. Preliminary evaluation of effects on recognition, attitudes and help-seeking behaviours indicated that such public courses might be useful in improving mental health literacy levels (Kitchener & Jorm, 2002). A unique feature of the National Plan in New Zealand (The Mental Health Commission, 1998) which was devised as part of the Blueprint for Mental Health Services to combat stigma and discrimination associated with mental illness, is the involvement of the indigenous communities. It mirrors the programme envisioned in Canada that seeks to empower the Aboriginal communities to build on their cultural resources to develop programmes and services that meet their own physical, mental, and spiritual needs.

In his very resourceful report, Arboleda-Flórez (2001) notes that initiatives from the developing world include the grand alliance of citizens and organisations involved with mental health in El Salvador under the auspices of the National Mental Health Council. Though disrupted by the massive earthquake that devastated the country at the beginning of 2001, the groundwork accomplished in the establishment of the Council gave impetus for a massive mobilisation of national forces to set up community grassroots activities, determined to immunise the people against the effects of the catastrophe on mental health, the prevention of panic reactions especially among young children, and the immediate treatment of those already affected by post-traumatic stress reactions. An alliance of mental health professionals/organisations with government bureaucracies and educational establishments across the country led to the development of in-field training for nurses, teachers, and other local community human resources personnel, much of which was carried out in the rubble of the devastating earthquake. Arboleda-Flórez concluded that the decisive emergency mental health action of El Salvador and the impact that it has had on demystifying mental illness and emotional problems, hence decreasing stigma, is one of the lessons on the potential of the human person for decisive action where there is the will and despite minimal resources.

In Tajikistan where there is a hostile and fearful attitude toward psychiatric illness, a national NGO (The Union of Mental Health Support) was created in 1998 to prevent stigma related to psychiatric disorders and to provide appropriate measures and assistance to psychiatric institutions. A survey was conducted to assess community attitudes toward mental illness and psychosocial distress with a view to using the result in the design of community education and awareness campaign (Baibabayev, Cunningham, & de Jong, 2000). The parliament passed a new law, abrogating the existing one that allowed the abuse of psychiatry for political purposes. In Slovakia, where the euphoria following the change of political leadership was dimmed by unrealised expectations which resulted in a sense of hopelessness in the population, stigma of persons with mental illness remains one of the three major mental health concerns. Reform efforts have intensified with an increased interest in the field of psychiatry among young physicians (Breier, 2000).

Recognising the importance of giving persons with psychosocial and intellectual disabilities a voice, especially as the 'experts' in their situations who should therefore be key partners among all stakeholders within the mental health sector, the South African Mental Health Movement (SAMHAM) was established by the South African Federation of Mental Health (SAFMH) in 2007. The body focuses on the development of an effective and representative national network of persons with psychosocial and intellectual disabilities. SAFMH aims to build on this as a national structure for ongoing empowerment of persons with psychosocial and intellectual disabilities and to raise awareness through contact-based education at the community level across the state.

SAMHAM forms a key component of the South African Federation for Mental Health's ongoing efforts to improve the reporting of human rights violations, as it provides the platform through which persons with psychosocial and intellectual disabilities and their families can report and escalate human rights violations from community-based settings across South Africa. It empowers persons with psychosocial and intellectual disabilities through enlightenment campaigns across the country. It is also involved in the drafting and reviewing of policies and legislation and is committed to ensuring that the rights of persons with psychosocial and intellectual disabilities are protected within South African legal frameworks.

International fellowships of people like Rotary International also identify with the anti-stigma campaigns. In 1996, Rotary International inaugurated *Erase the Stigma,* a campaign to educate American business leaders about the truths and misconceptions of severe mental illness. Sub-Saharan Africa and more of the developing world, with less developed mental health system, poor health outcomes, health inequalities and disparities needs more of these structures of advocacy that could draw from the effective activities of established agencies worldwide.

A Multi-dimensional Approach

It is unlikely that any one stigma-reduction intervention will effectively reduce stigmatising attitudes in everyone. A multidimensional approach based on evidence-based targeted interventions should include: primary prevention of disease, mental health education with experiential content, advocacy for social policies, and legislation that promote integration, cultural competency in care, and the engagement of the users' social network.

Broad approaches to increase mental health literacy may not be as effective as would specifically focused interventions among particular groups and on specific beliefs and attitudes. Anti-stigma campaigns may only prove successful if they take into account the complexity of the stigma process and if they are tailored to impact those defining components of stigma; cognitions, emotions and behaviours. There is also need to target specific mental disorders. As there are cultural dimensions to stigma, steps taken to combat stigma need also to be contextualised. They need to target providers at pre-service health education, in-service training, and in ongoing practice, enhancing their skills to engage people with psychiatric challenges. Identifying the origin of stigmatising attitudes in childhood or adolescence will help early interventions.

These stigma-reduction strategies do not always operate in isolation from one another. An advocate might educate media groups while protesting a stigmatising image of mental illness. A consumer group might recruit a person with mental illness to present an educational programme. Periodic longitudinal studies could help in the assessment of the impact of the interventions that have been introduced and also to determine the trends in public attitudes towards mental illness.

Part II

Barriers to Mental Healthcare

Introduction

Mental illness is charaterised by a clinically significant disturbance in an individual's cognition, emotion regulation, or behaviour, which reflects a dysfunction in the psychological, biological, or developmental processes underlying mental functioning (American Psychiatric Association, 2013). Mental disorders constitute risk factors for many health problems and are associated with distress, disability, increased risk of suffering pain, an important loss of freedom, or death. They create a substantial burden for affected individuals in terms of personal suffering and lifetime lost productivity. They also strain families in terms of a crippling burden of care and impact wider society in terms of the drain on resources.

Studies estimate that 792 million people live with a mental disorder, which is approximately one in ten people globally (10.7%) (Ritchie & Roser, 2018). Epidemiological findings suggest that almost 50% of the population will experience at least one mental disorder in their lifetime, and at least 25% have suffered from a mental disorder in a given year (Andrade et al., 2000). The global burden of mental illness accounts for 32·4% of years lived with disability (YLDs) and 13·0% of disability-adjusted life-years (DALYs). These place mental illness a comfortable first in the global burden of disease when measured by YLDs, and level with cardiovascular and circulatory diseases in terms of DALYs (Vigo, Thornicroft, & Atun, 2016). It was projected that common mental disorders would disable more people than complications arising from AIDS, heart disease, traffic accidents and wars combined by 2020 (Ngui, Khasakhala, Ndetei, & Roberts, 2010).

Such a disturbing trajectory notwithstanding, the mental health needs of people do not translate into seeking or receiving professional help, even when help is free (Corrigan, 2004; Ware, Manning, Duan, Wells, & Newhouse, 1984). Studies have consistently found that, even after clear-cut signs of psychotic disorders are developed, on average, it takes over a year before assessment and treatment are received (Black, Peters, Rui, Whitehorn, & Kopala, 2001; Compton, Kaslow, & Walker, 2004;

Johannessen et al., 2001). Delays of more than ten years are common if intervention is not made in the first year of the onset of mental illness (WHO/ICPE, 2000; Wang, Berglund, Olfson, & Kessler, 2004). Generally, 35–50% of people with a serious mental disorder in developed countries fail to receive treatment within one year, but the figure is doubled to 76.3–85.4% in developing countries (Demyttenaere et al., 2004; Wang et al., 2007).

Studies observe a disparity in access and service utilisation between ethnic and mainstream populations with the former underperforming. Such patterns are observed in many ethnic groups in a range of settings: the Punjabi in the UK (Bhui, Bhugra, Goldberg, Dunn, & Desai, 2001), Hispanic and Asian groups in the USA (Sue, 1977), and the Vietnamese in Australia (Phan, 2000). Whereas 16.6% of White adults received mental health services in the US in 2011, only 7.6% of Blacks, 7.3% of Hispanics, and 6.5% of Asians received any treatment (Corrigan, Druss, & Perlick, 2014). Studies also indicate that ethnic minority clients tend to terminate counselling at the rate of more than 50% after only one contact with a therapist, which is in marked contrast to the less than 30% termination rate among White clients (Sue, Sue, & Sue, 1997).

It was projected that mental disorders would account for as much as 18% of the disease conditions in Africa by 2020 (World Health Organisation WHO, 2001b). This is notwithstanding the high burden of communicable, maternal, perinatal, and nutrition-related diseases. A number of studies indicate that the utilisation rates for mental health services by Africans are disproportionately low compared to the burden of potentially treatable problems (Gaines, 1998; Kamya, 2001; Wong, 1997). The proportion of those with mental health needs receiving formal mental healthcare in Nigeria over 12 months was as low as 1.6% (Wang et al., 2007). Indeed, the under-utilisation of mental health facilities has been considered to be behind the previously held notion that Africans as a group have a lesser need for mental health services than do Caucasians (Vaughn & Holloway, 2009).

As delays in seeking help for mental health problems lead to poorer outcomes (Adeosun, Adegbohun, Adewumi, & Jeje, 2013), identifying the potential barriers to mental healthcare will be instrumental for decisive interventions. This section explores the ideological and instrumental barriers that impede access to mental health services, especially in low- and middle-income countries with sub-Saharan Africa and Nigeria as case studies. More pertinently, the section robustly interrogates the factors that influence health-seeking behaviour and compliance in migrant groups. The insights and recommendations should enable health systems to ensure equity of access and equality, especially given the growing concerns about inequities in health for Black, Asian and Minority Ethnic (BAME) groups.

7 Help-Seeking Determinants and Ideological Barriers

The Sociocultural Context

Culture is a social context in which people share social norms, beliefs, values, language and institutions (Guerra & Jagers, 1998). It provides a cognitive map of unwritten rules for living (Leininger & McFarland, 2002) and a framework for interpreting and giving meaning to personal experiences (Lindisfarne, 1998). Thus, the culture of a people is a model for human behaviour as people generally act in ways that correspond to cultural influences and expectations. Culturally constructed beliefs function as a prism in perceiving mental health issues and shaping pathways for help-seeking (Leong & Lau, 2001; Tabora & Flaskerud, 1997). People can feel 'trapped' within the values of tradition which affects perceptions of mental health issues and may inhibit willingness to engage with services (Gilbert, Gilbert, & Sanghera, 2004; Sen, 2001).

Arab women, for instance, can feel obliged to operate within a set of norms of family and community honour that can override personal concerns (Kassam, 1997). Living in a society that is both collectivist and paternalistic, these women see no acknowledged legitimisation for deviating from the traditional path. In these cultures, women can perceive themselves as 'carriers' of family honour, requiring them to modulate their actions so as not to dishonour or bring shame upon the family. Exploring psychological distress and self-harm, Chew-Graham and colleagues (2002) found that 'Izzat' (a set of norms of family and community honour in Asia) could be used to reinforce a woman's subordinate role in family life and to coerce women into remaining silent about their problems.

Asian students were found to be far more focused on external shame (what others think) and reflected shame (shame they can bring to others, e.g. family), than non-Asian students. Yet they do not suffer any less from internal shame (Gilbert et al., 2007). Studies of Asian and African immigrants in Western cultures also show that the more closely people adhered to their ethnic, cultural values, the less likely they were to seek professional psychological help for mental health concerns (Essandoh, 1995; Hamid, Simmonds, & Bowles, 2009).

As Cauce and colleagues (2002) noted, when salient and valued social norms are incongruent with formal service use, individuals will inevitably be influenced not to seek help. For instance, sociocultural norms such as a high regard for saving face characteristic of the Igbo culture of south-eastern Nigeria may deviate from the basic principles of formal treatment such as disclosure and may inevitably translate into underutilisation of professional mental health services. This is reflected in 74.9% of the respondents in the case study of south-eastern Nigeria (Ikwuka, 2016) indicating that, before discussing the mental health problem of someone close to them, they must be sure they are talking to someone they can trust with a secret. Similarly, 61.3% of the respondents believed that problems such as mental illness are better handled privately because of the shame they could bring. Mental illness is a taboo in this culture, and discussions about it are treated with utmost confidentiality beyond the formality of data protection. The mental health crisis of a family member is among the things that are discussed in hushed tones, and it could be very unnerving to be openly identified with a psychiatrist or psychiatric hospitalisation.

Drummond and colleagues (2011) discovered that shame was a significant factor dissuading West African refugee women in Australia from seeking help for mental illness. A further cultural twist to the finding was that the more educated among the women felt more shame being associated with mental illness than the less educated. This surprised the Australian researchers presumably because they had supposed that education would have a moderating effect on the sense of shame. But this is not the case in a cultural setting where social conformity is achieved through the use of 'shaming' (including public booing) as a sanction against culturally unacceptable behaviour (Nzewi, 1989). Thus, in their socialisation, shame is associated with deviance such that 'higher status' and more educated individuals would be much more wary of a situation that would bring them shame. Until psychiatric illness is normalised in such regions, to be culturally appropriate, services must proceed with the utmost confidentiality.

Moreover, the dichotomy between the unitary African and dualistic Western conceptions of reality could be reflected in the people's help-seeking behaviour. As Lambo (1978) observed, the African world-view does not discriminate between the living and non-living, conscious and unconscious, natural and supernatural. These pairs which are conceived of as opposites in the West are realised as unities in Africa. For instance, there is a deep sense of reverence for ancestors, who are believed to intervene actively in the affairs of the living. Such a vision of reality, whereby the seen and the unseen dynamically interrelate, contrasts with the dualism of the West, such that an experience like hearing of voices, which could easily be pathologised as a hallucination in the latter, could, for instance, be welcomed in the former as communication with ancestors – a spiritual gift (Furnham & Igboaka, 2007; Nwoko, 2009). A similar experience is reported of indigenes in the Pacific island of Bali who believe that to become a traditional healer, one has to experience an episode quite similar to psychosis which, when resolved without active treatment, is confirmation that an individual has been selected super-naturally to be a healer and hence endowed with special ability and powers (Stephen & Suryani, 2000). Against such backgrounds, Dinos and colleagues (2017) contend that for experiences to be labelled as psychotic, they need to be unexplainable from a cultural perspective or from what would be considered acceptable in a local context and by the peer group of the patient.

The unitary vision of reality is also consistent with the relatively greater somatisation of distress reported in sub-Saharan Africa whereby psychological problems present in physical symptoms, a tendency associated with seeking treatment for mental health problems in the general medical rather than the psychiatric sector (Alegria et al., 1991; Corrigan, Druss & Perlick, 2014). Ranguram and Weiss (2004) considered that generally, physical illnesses tend to be associated with lesser stigma than mental illnesses, and this may contribute to a high presentation of somatic complaints in patients with underlying mental illnesses in areas where there is low mental health literacy. Here, doctors are consulted mostly for physical symptoms, hence the undiagnosed persistence of psychological distress.

Russell and colleagues (2008) found that a greater number of im-migrant students presenting with more severe mental health symptoms felt the need to seek help from medical health professionals rather than counselling services. Compared with American students, who tend to experience stress as anxiety and/or depression (Aubrey, 1991), foreign students struggle with the discrimination between emotional distress and somatic illnesses and may attribute their problems to organic processes (Flaskerud, 1986; Russell, Thomson, & Rosenthal, 2008). This could lead to a delay in psychiatric help-seeking.

Somatisation may also be indicative of a lack of emotional competence (the ability to identify, understand, describe and manage emotions in an effective manner) which has equally been linked with poor help-seeking behaviour (Ciarrochi & Deane 2001). Nwokocha (2010) observed that language plays an important role in how a person communicates mental health concerns and that a person's inability to express their symptoms, or a practitioner's inability to understand symptom conceptualisation can influence and even change the attitude of the mental health provider. On the other hand, it was also observed that some clinicians from Western cultures fail to recognise or appreciate the seriousness of somatised symptoms expressed in some of the immigrant cultures and, as a result, not all the symptoms are being addressed (Nwokocha, 2005).

The Conceptualisation of Disease

All psychiatric categories are culturally construed (Littlewood, 1996). Mental illness assumes cultural meaning which shapes the way people perceive, suffer and cope with it. Demonstrating contextual variation in help-seeking behaviours, a pioneering study that used identical data collection processes and instruments in Egypt, Kuwait, Palestine, and among Israeli Arabs, found that respondents within the various countries, based on nationality, gender and level of education, varied in terms of recognition of personal need, beliefs about mental health problems, and the use of traditional healing methods versus modern approaches to psychiatric therapy (Al-Krenawi, Graham, Al-Bedah, Kadri, & Sehwail, 2009).

Asian respondents who subscribed to Western models of illness had a more positive disposition towards seeking Western biomedical psychiatric care, while those that held supernatural beliefs had more negative attitudes towards biomedical psychiatric care (Fung & Wong, 2007). The appeal of non-biomedical models of care was mostly informed by their compliance with the judgments of the patients pertaining to the meaning and nature of health and illness, their world views, and their religious beliefs (Chadda, Agarwal, Chandra, & Raheja, 2001). Significant dilemmas arise when patients' explanatory models (EMs) differ significantly from the dominant standardised explanations offered by psychiatric research, such that patients' treatment preferences are not easily fulfilled (Dinos et al., 2017).

It has been observed that factors that lead patients from ethnic backgrounds to feel alienated from mainline biomedical health clinics and providers include different understandings of mental illness (Martin, 2009; Vera et al., 1998), and ignorance of culturally different symptom expression (Hunter & Schmidt, 2010; Tófoli, Andrade, & Fortes, 2011). It is also observed that a lack of bilingual and bicultural professionals creates cultural and linguistic barriers that prevent immigrants from obtaining proper mental healthcare (Spector, 1996).

Angel and Thoits (1987) reported how the failure to consider how Mexican culture shapes the self-reports of physiological symptoms of Mexican Americans resulted in serious errors in the findings of epidemiologic studies, which underrated the illness for individuals at greater risk of poor health. In *Crazy like Us*, Watters (2010) cites cross-cultural examples demonstrating how the global 'imposition' of Western conceptualisations of mental illness has potentially altered how distress is manifested or introduced barriers to recovery. Following the tsunami that struck Sri Lanka in 2004, Watters recalls how Gaithri Fernando, a young Sri Lankan clinical psychologist, resident in the US, who witnessed the tsunami, observed that unlike the PTSD symptomatology which informed the intervention introduced by the emergency services from the West, Sri Lankans were much more likely to report physical symptoms (somatisation). They did not report pathological reactions to trauma in line with the internal states (anxiety, fear, numbing etc.) of the PTSD symptom checklist but the negative consequences of the disaster were evaluated in terms of the damage they did to social relationships.

Regier and colleagues (1988) note that the general public in the West are more likely to recognise mood rather than somatic symptoms (of depression), which is different in Arabic, Asian and African cultures where somatisation is a common expression of mental illness and description of mood changes are rare. Psycho-physiological complaints such as depression are often subjectively represented by the African as bodily sensations including: a sensation of heaviness in the brain, a feeling that the belly is bloated with water, heat in the head and body, the sense that the heart is melting and wants to fly away, a sensation of worms crawling all over the body, a lump in the throat or burning sensations in the body (Okhomina & Ebie, 1973). For similar pathologies, the West would report feeling worthless, losing interest in usual activities, being unable to start or finish anything and suicidal ideation (Idemudia, 2004).

There are also cultural variations in the indicators of good or poor mental health. For instance, Earle (1998) reported that, compared to a Caucasian sample, American Indians considered attributes such as having visions or living according to the dictates of spirits as good mental health indicators. Suan and Taylor (1990) also found that Japanese-American college students rated characteristics such as untrustworthiness, exhibiting poor interpersonal relations and a negative personality as stronger indicators of poor individual mental health than Caucasian-American college students.

Labels of health conditions such as 'schizophrenia' and 'mental illness' are also understood differently across cultures. For example, a survey in Germany found that 79.6% of the public believe that people with schizophrenia suffer from split or multiple personalities (Gaebel, Baumann, Witte, & Zaeske, 2002) compared to only 47.2% in a Canadian public sample (Stuart & Arboleda-Flórez, 2001b). A cross-national study found that 31.6% of a German sample linked schizophrenia with split personality compared with only 2.0% of a Russian sample (Schomerus, Kenzin, Borsche, Matschinger & Angermeyer, 2007). Angermeyer and colleagues (2004) found that labelling of a schizophrenia vignette was associated with perceived dangerousness in a sample of the German public but not in Russian or Mongolian samples. Common mental disorders (CMDs) such as depression and anxiety also vary considerably across cultural and social contexts in terms of prevalence, symptomatology, treatment and help-seeking behaviour (Kirmayer & Jarvis, 2006).

Studies in India show that CMDs are not understood as mental illness, rather, 'mental illness' refers mostly to psychotic disorders (Patel et al., 1997). Similarly, though symptom severity is associated with help-seeking (Biddle, Gunnel, Sharp & Donovan, 2004), the Nigerian general public also conceives mental illness in terms of severe psychotic disorders (madness) and associate mental illness with vagrancy (Atilola & Olayiwola, 2011; Ewhrudjakpor, 2010a; Igbinomwanhia, James, & Omoaregba, 2013). Such extreme conceptualisation of mental illness not only connotes 'insanity' which requires hospitalisation/detention and is mostly irremediable but also results in strong stigmatisation of mental illness in general, which is a leading barrier to help-seeking. It could lead to reluctance to acknowledge distress as a mental health problem and a corresponding disinclination to seek help. It could also imply potential misunderstanding and undermining of other non-psychotic disorders for which help may therefore not be sought. For example, a condition such as Attention Deficit Hyperactivity Disorder (ADHD) could be interpreted as delinquency in children and handled punitively. Possibly, it is with such a notion that clients with a subtle onset of mental illness, for example, those praying continuously, were not recognised in time as suffering from mental illness in a South African study (Mkize & Uys, 2004).

In an earlier Ethiopian study, only 12% of respondents considered alcoholism a serious mental illness. Sixty-six per cent recommended no treatment for it or sending the patient to prison (Khandelwal & Workneh, 1986). Idioms of distress (characteristic modes of expressing distress) are also mostly based on cultural and contextual peculiarities (Nichter, 1981). Cultural determination of distress is such that Angel and Thoits (1987) suggested that the clinical facts of the disease are only loosely related to the subjective experience of the illness.

The foregoing indicates that different conceptions of mental health significantly exist and may be misunderstood by therapists, particularly those of different backgrounds from their clients. It underscores the need to analyse and understand particular manifestations of distress in context. It further indicates that determining the conceptualisation of mental health could help in understanding the differences in attitudes towards mental illness, symptom presentation and help-seeking behaviours, thereby helping to unravel the reasons for underutilisation of mental health services. Institutional racism and cultural misunderstandings of idioms of distress, based on ignorance, prejudice and racial stereotyping, undermine diagnostic accuracy and ultimately lead to the pathologisation of culture and culturally adaptive behaviours (Dinos et al., 2017). Culturally sensitive clinical approaches, based on the exploration of explanatory models during assessment and treatment, could be an effective way to deal with the complexity of service users' needs. Knowledge of explanatory models (EMs) can be a powerful tool to strengthen the therapeutic alliance between health professionals and patients, maximise collaboration, improve communication, make more accurate diagnoses for effective culturally appropriate interventions and ultimately enhance clinical outcomes.

Cultural (In)appropriateness of Care

Questions have been raised regarding the cultural appropriateness of biomedical psychiatric care (Vaillant, 2012). The model may be perceived as having strong historical and epistemological anchors to Western Europe and North America. An ethnocentric view of psychopathology can limit our understanding of disorders in general, and the pathways through which non-Westerners can approach treatment (Gaines, 1998; Idemudia, 2004). Moreover, the heritage of relations between the dominant White and ethnic minorities means that there are profound reasons why some people will be suspicious of what is seen to be a White-dominated service. For instance, for most post-colonial peoples, there may be politically embedded ambivalence towards modern mental health services.

Perceived efficacy notwithstanding, mental health services are identified as part of the colonial process and as having a limited cultural sensitivity towards minority groups (Al-Krenawi & Graham, 2011). Antipathy towards biomedical psychiatric care and the popularisation of the traditional model could therefore be expressive of a nationalistic mindset and a pro-indigenisation policy whereby traditional medicine enjoys popular media coverage, and traditional healers openly challenge the utility of Western medicine and gain popularity, especially amongst the poor (Uzochukwu & Onwujekwe, 2004). Mental health services represent Western culture insofar as they may be perceived as undermining native values, which may hinder their acceptance.

The process of psychiatric diagnosis (the International Classification Systems ICD) has been criticised for assuming that diagnostic categories have the same meaning when carried over to a new cultural context (Kleinman, 1977, 1987). Prior to ICD-10, which acknowledged that there are exceptions to the presumed universality of psychiatric diagnoses, culture-specific disorders such as brain fag syndrome (a concept initially used almost exclusively in West Africa to depict a condition often associated with male students and generally presenting as vague somatic symptoms, depression and difficulty concentrating) and *koro* (a form of genital retraction anxiety which presents in parts of Asia) tended to be subsumed into such established diagnostic categories as delusional disorder (Crozier, 2011).

Minas and Cohen (2007) note that a major impediment to the development of an effective, appropriate, affordable and equitable mental healthcare delivery system is the lack of evidence-based information on which kinds of mental health systems are appropriate and effective in varying political, social and economic contexts. Bolman (1968) had earlier observed that one of the major obstacles in the development of mental health services in the developing non-Western world is the difficulty in making culturally and linguistically specific adaptations of Western scientific approaches. This dissonance is immediately evident in the observation in the region that public beliefs regarding the causes of mental disorders, and the effectiveness of various treatments, differed significantly from those of mental health professionals and that, despite their knowledge base, the cultural values of health professionals still affected their attitudes towards their care of persons with mental illness (Afolayan & Okpemuza, 2010; Magliano, Fiorillo, de Rosa, Malangone & Maj, 2004).

Sociocultural differences between the provider and consumer engender systematic biases and misunderstandings that hamper communication (Betancourt & Maina, 2007). Conflicts between traditional and Western cultural values lead to high dropout rates and underutilisation of community mental health resources (Hsu, 2003). Cultural mistrust or misunderstanding between therapists and clients is often used to explain the existence and perpetuation of racial and ethnic disparities in mental health help-seeking and utilisation (Nickerson, Helms, & Terrell, 1994; Suite, La Bril, Primm, & Harrison-Ross, 2007).

The therapeutic procedure of the biomedical model of care could also be adjudged culturally inappropriate in the traditional sub-Saharan African context where the ability to make quick and accurate diagnoses leading to timely intervention is intrinsic to the paradigm of an expert, for instance, a specialist or consultant. As Nzewi (1989) noted, extensive and prolonged interrogations are viewed with displeasure and usually generate a lack of confidence in the therapeutic process. Thus the bureaucracy and seemingly superfluous discourse characteristic of biomedical care and psychological therapies would be met with serious disappointment. In times of crises, it would appear inappropriate to be kept waiting.

This was somewhat reflected in a study by Keynejad (2008) which explored what inhibits ethnic minority groups from accessing mental health services in London. The study reported that ethnic minorities with multiple needs felt they were always being referred from one agency to another while some felt that any waiting list they would be put on would be so long that it would not be worth seeking help. They considered the seemingly dragging protocols as evidence of lack of seriousness on the part of the system. A study that investigated the factors militating against keeping an appointment for initial screening at a community mental health centre found a positive relationship between the length of time that patients have to wait for the first appointment and the rate of failure to keep an appointment ('no-show' rate) (Peeters & Bayer, 1999). The most prevalent reasons for 'no-show' were: being on the waiting list, lack of motivation, and lack of resolution of the mental health problem. The patient's disposition has also been demonstrated to facilitate the therapeutic process (Ogrodniczuk, Joyce, & Piper, 2005).

Conversant with the sense of urgency for results in these cultures, traditional and spiritual healers go to the length of anticipating the complaints of the clients, thereby earning their confidence and disposing them positively towards the therapeutic process. Nzewi (1989) reported on the experience of an anxious mother of a teenage girl with hysterical paralysis of the legs. As she started to give a lengthy description of her daughter's problems, after a period of seeming inattention by the native healer, he dramatically commanded "Stop! How dare you try to seek for the all-seeing eyes and think for the all-knowing mind? You have come to me, let me tell you your problems because I know what they are already." After some theatricals *"anwansi"*, he proceeded to put together what appeared to be a correct picture of the patient's problems to the awe and amazement of his audience.

However, in this art of mind games, he already had some idea about the symptoms of this particular illness, and all he needed was some clue from the discloser, and he could proceed to make a quick 'authoritative' diagnosis in order to gain the immediate confidence of the clients. While the *anwansi* means of gaining clients' confidence by the native healer could raise ethical questions, the idea underscores the need for therapists and biomedical care providers in these contexts to demonstrate both professional and cultural competence and adapt these to achieve a therapeutic alliance with clients, especially in a culture where the reputation of the care provider decisively shapes help-seeking behaviour (Asenso-Okyere, 1998).

Sociocultural norms also influence consumers' preferences for setting and achieving treatment goals and outcomes (Hwang, Myers, Abe-Ku, & Ting, 2008). For instance, while in the biomedical model, based on individualistic Western culture, the major indicator of recovery rests on overcoming disabilities to meet occupational goals – achieving independence (Davidson, Rakfeldt, & Strauss, 2010; Liberman, 2008), in the communalistic African context, the ultimate end to which the therapeutic process would aim is to help make a deviant character conform (to social norms) – a behavioural goal. In the traditional communalistic African culture, where independence is not an ideal but could actually be pathologised, the community (family) naturally assumes the roles of 'hands' and 'feet' for the disabled person who banks on this support. This perhaps explains why occupational therapy is not popular in the region with a median rate of 0.01 occupational therapists to 100,000 population (WHO, 2011). This also indicates that the recognition of individual distress as a marker of mental illness will be less prominent than social indicators in this culture.

Lack of cultural competence and appropriate intervention strategies on the part of treatment providers constitute the most formidable barriers to mental health service use by non-Western cultures (Takeuchi, Bui, & Kim, 1993). They are considered to make services less user-friendly for patients from Non-English-Speaking Backgrounds (NESB) (Mitchell, Malak, & Small, 1998; Tobin, 2000) and could result in the pattern whereby ethnic minority groups may have higher rates of mental illnesses, lower rates of general referral and treatment, but higher rates of compulsory treatment and forensic service contact (Dinos, Stevens, Serfaty, Weich, & King, 2014; Keating & Robertson, 2004; National Institute for Mental Health in England, 2003). The American Psychiatric Association (2018) has indeed acknowledged that the disparity does not stem from a greater prevalence rate or severity of illness in ethnic minority groups but from a lack of culturally competent care and from ethnic minority groups receiving less or poor-quality care.

Cultural appropriateness of service is the most significant predictor of attitudes towards seeking professional help for mental illness as was found in a survey of five ethnic minority groups (Fung & Wong, 2007). White women felt more comfortable with predominantly White healthcare providers than their Black and Hispanic counterparts (Doornbos, Zandee, DeGroot, & De Maagd-Rodriguez, 2013). This is consistent with previous findings where depressed African-American women had a deep mistrust of the healthcare system as a 'White system' (Nicolaidis et al., 2010). The observation that Hispanics, Native Americans, Blacks and Asian-Americans have a tendency for early termination of psychotherapeutic treatment and also average fewer sessions than Whites (Sue, Sue, & Sue, 1997) may not be unconnected with the possibility that therapists fail to provide culturally responsive forms of treatment.

Communication problems due to language barriers have equally been implicated in non-attendance at outpatient clinics (Stern, Cottrell, & Holmes, 1990). The more populations become diverse, the more the need for culturally competent and appropriate healthcare services. It is observed that the relatively more positive attitude of the American population towards mental health services is traceable to the ubiquity of the facilities (Al-Darmaki, 2003). As culture shapes the patients' view of their mental health and their service use, as well as that of the care providers and the service system with respect to diagnosis and treatment, cultural differences must be accounted for to ensure that all receive mental healthcare tailored to their needs.

Carrillo and colleagues (1999) note that for mental health service delivery to be effective and efficient, key socio-cultural issues that are relevant to the provision of culturally responsive services must be considered for example salience of family and social support, importance of religion or spirituality, stress of migration, barriers of language or literacy, and impact of socioeconomic factors. Significant dislocation from one's culture, even in the process of therapy can be maladaptive (Chen, Benet-Martinez, & Bond, 2008). Thus, the therapist must, of necessity, be an ecologist; realising that his patient has desires, beliefs, habits and patterns of associations, all of which influence his health.

To make for culturally competent therapy, the British Psychological Association's Division of Clinical Psychology recommended adherence to guidelines stipulating that all clinical psychologists must contribute to the direct provision of psychological therapies which take into account cultural differences, the impact of racism on psychological health, and the specific needs of Black and Minority Ethnic people (British Psychological Association, 1998). Furthermore, following a landmark case in ethnic minority mental health whereby David Bennett, a 38-year-old African-Caribbean man, died on October 30, 1998, in a medium secure psychiatric unit after being restrained by staff, many issues surrounding cultural and racial equality in mental healthcare that needed resolving in the UK National Health Service (NHS) were highlighted. The government responded in 2005 with a plan for Delivering Race Equality (DRE) in mental healthcare (Department of Health, 2005) which aimed at more appropriate and responsive services, community engagement and better information.

Among other things, DRE aimed that, by 2010, mental health services in the UK would be characterised by:

1   Less fear of mental health services among Black, Asian and Minority Ethnic (BAME) communities and service users
2   A reduction in the rate of admission of people from BAME communities to psychiatric inpatient units
3   A reduction in the disproportionate rates of compulsory detention of BAME service users in inpatient units
4   A reduction in the use of seclusion in BAME groups
5   More BAME service users reaching self-reported states of recovery
6   A reduction in the ethnic disparities found in prison populations
7   A more balanced range of effective therapies such as peer support services and psychotherapeutic and counselling treatments, as well as pharmacological interventions that are culturally appropriate and effective
8   A more active role for BAME communities and BAME service users in the training of professionals, in the development of mental health policy and in the planning and provision of services
9   A workforce and organisation capable of delivering appropriate and responsive mental health services to BAME communities

While the timetables of the NHS workforce are now replete with mandatory training programmes in cultural competence (Dinos, 2015), the widespread cultural adaptation of existing evidence-based interventions (EBIs) is still to be achieved (Dinos et al., 2017). The US Surgeon General Report (DHHS, 2001) noted that minorities typically delay seeking treatment, and similarly encouraged the development of ethnic-specific programmes that match patients to therapists. Furthermore, following the influx of immigrants to the United States from 1990 to 2000, the US social service and mental health systems equally generated new services, appropriate sensitivity and interventions for the nation's newest immigrants (Foster, 2001).

Faced with the more challenging aspects of other cultural models such as spirit-based belief, the Western therapist will require openness to the guidance of non-Western colleagues and patients, in order to overcome stereotypical responses (Dixon, 2008; Nyagua & Harris, 2007). Cultural competency in service delivery also demands that while the "universals" in mental health pathologies are promoted, healthcare providers also need to be conversant with the cultural anthropology of the people they serve. This is deserving of priority in the curriculum of trainee health workers and therapists.

Lin (1991) advocates for close adherence to the tenet of cultural relativity, together with efforts in obtaining relevant information regarding the meaning and consequences of the symptoms in the patient's cultural context. However, he equally observes that excessive preoccupation with cultural influences in psychiatric symptom presentation may conversely lead to the underestimation of psychopathology. He, therefore, calls for adequate attention to the universal aspects of psychopathology in counterbalancing such a tendency (as cited in Thomas, 2008).

Mental Health Literacy

Mental health literacy is the knowledge and understanding about mental disorders which aid their recognition, management or prevention (Jorm, 2000). Studies indicate that mental health literacy is positively associated with a disposition to seek mental healthcare while lack of knowledge and information, leading to negative stereotypes of mental illness in the community serve as critical barriers to service utilisation (Gulliver, Griffiths, & Christensen, 2010; Larson & Corrigan, 2008; Rüsch, Evans-Lacko, Henderson, Flach, & Thornicroft, 2011). Lack of mental health literacy could also act as an impediment to early recognition of a disorder (Hugo, Boshoff, Traut, Zungu-Dirwayi, & Stein, 2003). Members of the public generally demonstrate a lack of mental health literacy (Angermeyer & Dietrich, 2006; Magliano et al., 2004).

Epidemiological research suggests that as many as half the people with diagnoses of such conditions as schizophrenia and bipolar disorder are unaware of their condition (Kessler et al., 2001). Lack of knowledge regarding the availability of effective treatment, and where and how to access it, also leads to underutilisation of biomedical mental healthcare (Gulbinat, Manderscheid, Baingana et al., 2004; Hugo et al., 2003; Thornicroft, 2008). It is revealing that even medical students demonstrated poor awareness of existing services (Chew-Graham, Rogers, & Yassin, 2003). Results from a study that compared international students' awareness and use of counselling services with their levels of academic stress found that those who were aware of the availability of counselling services reported significantly lower levels of academic stress than those unaware of the availability of those services (Nina, 2009).

Beliefs concerning psychiatric treatment itself could also constitute a barrier towards seeking treatment. Some people believe that psychiatric hospitals are for lunatics; people who are violent, rejected by society, and subsequently locked away (Budman, Lipson, & Meleis, 1992). A community study of attitudes to mental illness in Nigeria showed that more than half of the respondents thought that people with mental illness should not receive treatment from normal health facilities owing to the communities' attribution of dangerousness to the patients (Gureje, Lasebikan, Ephraim-Oluwanuga, Olley, & Kola, 2005). The Nigerian public generally has poor knowledge about mental disorders, the availability of mental health services and effective treatment outcomes (Jack-Ide & Uys, 2013).

In the case study of south-eastern Nigeria (Ikwuka, 2016), while 63.8% of the respondents thought that mixed causal factors for mental illness meant confusion regarding where to seek help, half of the respondents (50.7%) categorically stated that they would not be sure of where to seek help. Moreover, 65.9% of respondents thought that mental health does not exist along a continuum, that people are either 'mad' or not 'mad'. Such dichotomous understanding of mental health does not encourage help-seeking, especially when symptoms are not debilitating. This was demonstrated in a study with African Americans in the US where many said they did not think they were 'crazy', therefore they did not seek mental health services (Hines-Martin, Brown-Piper, Kim, & Malone, 2003). A similar mindset was reported by a community health worker in a Southern African survey: "We go out to visit these villages and sometimes we find people who feel that we are wasting their time because they believe that health only needs attention when it is giving problems" (Obioha & Molale, 2011).

Such notions are further reinforced in the Nigerian context where the gravity of psychiatric illness is judged on behavioural grounds, a conception corroborated by 81.3% of the respondents in the case study (Ikwuka, 2016) indicating that mental illness is recognisable only when the individual begins to 'misbehave'. Holding such idioms of distress could potentially delay help-seeking since overt behavioural symptoms could manifest belatedly, or even be entirely lacking in the course of a disorder. This is further reinforced in 50% of the respondents submitting that mental illness is not usually noticed in time. These underscore the observation by Mkize and Uys (2004) that, in the traditional African context, the social network assesses the severity of a person's sickness by the extent of the person's activity. If a sick person continues to work, then the sickness is minor. Sickness is considered serious, mostly when the patient is bedridden. Recognition of symptoms is the gateway to help-seeking, as action taken regarding sickness depends on whether the communities under study perceive the condition as a major health problem.

Furthermore, in this region, the sudden onset of psychotic conditions, which could come with bizarre symptoms and at the prime of life, usually destabilises the uninformed families. Fuelled by the deeply religious world-view of the people, such 'strange' occurrences logically attract supernatural attribution with the immediate response usually being recourse to the spiritual help pathway. Such conceptualisation could equally diminish the effectiveness of biomedical psychiatry. As Link and colleagues (1999) observe, cultural misconceptions about mental illness could lead to negative stereotypes of established systems of care and help-seeking, 2010).

Similarly, a common element in the African belief system is that mental and physical illness can also result from disequilibrium in the harmony between an individual and the cosmos. In spite of the cultural and ethnic diversity in Africa, there is a general belief that both physical and mental diseases could originate from various social and spiritual factors such as the breach of a taboo or custom, disturbances in social relations, hostile ancestral spirits, spirit/demonic possession, evil forces, sorcery, affliction by God or gods and natural causes (Betancourt, Green, & Carrillo, 2000; Idemudia, 2004; Okafor, 2009). Judgments of responsibility follow attributions of personal causality. There is, for instance, an observed increase in causally linking mental illness to the use of illicit drugs and alcohol in most of sub-Saharan Africa which are viewed negatively and linked to moral failings on the part of the user (Aghukwa, 2009a; Crabb, 2012). Reinforced by the strong belief of these societies in retributive justice, when mental illness is associated with self-destructive behaviour, sufferers could be condemned as paying for their 'sins', which risks non-medical treatment, discrimination, rejection and even maltreatment by the public including healthcare professionals.

Another important medium which demonstrates a lack of mental health literacy is pessimism regarding prognoses. Many Nigerians believe that mental illness is incurable and terminal (Aghukwa 2009b; Ewhrudjakpor, 2009). Entrenched pessimism regarding the course of mental illness is captured in a popular Igbo proverb *agwọsia onyeara, adighi agwọ ya ntamu* which literally translates that, however well a madman is cured, his tendency to soliloquise remains. In other words, full symptom remission is impossible. This view is endorsed by close to half of the respondents (46.4%) in the case study of south-eastern Nigeria (Ikwuka, 2016). Only 9% of doctors in a comparable south-western Nigerian study believed that mental illness could be cured (Adewuya & Oguntade, 2007). As beliefs about the effectiveness of treatment and services influence subsequent treatment behaviour (Dosreis et al., 2009), such myths of incurability could discourage help-seeking as futile – a waste of time and resources.

Most mental disorders can be effectively treated or managed, but having evidence-based treatments available is not enough if the public does not perceive biomedical psychiatric interventions as effective. Research has demonstrated that increasing public understanding of mental health conditions and awareness that effective treatment is available, is critical in improving help-seeking behaviour (Patel et al., 2007; Wang et al., 2007). Public health campaigns are therefore necessary to enlighten the public about the available treatments for mental health problems with promising results. Controlled evaluation showed that ten weeks after the presentations given by trained GPs, students' intentions to consult a GP for physical and psychological problems significantly increased and their barriers to engaging with a GP had significantly decreased (Wilson, Bignell, & Clancy, 2003).

Preliminary evaluation of mental health first-aid training courses for the general public also showed that such public courses might be useful in improving mental health literacy levels (Kitchener & Jorm, 2002). Education also helps in the normalisation of mental illness (see Chapter 6, Education), resulting in greater confidence in seeking help following de-stigmatisation. Improving mental health literacy in predominantly rural communities of developing societies could focus on changing attitudes such as self-reliance and the preference for informal help. As somatisation is a common idiom of distress in these cultures, efforts to enlighten the public about symptoms could be focused on the somatic presentation of underlying symptoms. Given that initial recognition and response to mental health problems generally takes place in the community, and the significant influence of the social networks in the help-seeking pathway, the family should be empowered with knowledge and the mechanism of referral. As the onset of psychosis can be unforeseen with unnerving symptoms, general awareness about the disorder could prepare people/families for the unexpected, making them more confident to make more rational decisions, especially in view of the pressure and confusion of unsolicited prescriptions from the social network.

Culture of Self-reliance

Culturally gendered roles may have implications for help-seeking. For instance, men are generally socialised to believe that power, dominance, competition and control are essential in proving one's masculinity (Robertson & Fitzgerald, 1992). Males are significantly less likely from an early age to report problems or seek help, due to a deep-seated need to appear in control and not to show vulnerability which is based on this traditional sex-role stereotyping and an ideology of self-reliance (Benenson & Koulnazarian, 2008; Elliot-Schmidt & Strong, 1997). In keeping with the traditional masculine gender role prescriptions, people who seek psychological services have been stereotyped as crazy, weak, or out of control (Corrigan, 2004).

In contrast to women, men may also associate formal help-seeking with a diminishment of their abilities to be strong providers and family leaders (Komiti, Judd, & Jackson, 2006; El-Islam 2000). Furthermore, men's traditionally advantaged social status, greater control and decision-making power, and higher income than women may make it difficult for them to accept a diagnosis of a potentially disabling condition such as a mental disorder, or to seek help for it (Judd, Komiti, & Jackson, 2008). This can lead to a preference for self coping, seeking help as a last resort, or reliance on informal, rather than formal services.

As noted by Uzochukwu and Onwujekwe (2004), self-diagnosis of illness is very common in the masculinist Igbo system of south-eastern Nigeria, though this could also be an adaptive response to the poor and inadequate mental health system. Furthermore, the strong traditional masculinity in this system demands that 'men should be men' – they should subdue their emotions. It is effeminate to shed tears. Hence, emotions which could be symptomatic and assist diagnosis could be stifled. One consequence of such masculinist disposition is the finding that men's mental conditions upon treatment entry are typically more serious (Smith, Tran, & Thompson, 2008), possibly owing to a belated presentation at mental health facilities.

Research also suggests that adolescents and young adults demonstrate the strongest tendencies for self-help in dealing with mental health difficulties (Gulliver et al., 2010; Rickwood, Deane, & Wilson, 2007). Such a stoic culture which avoids overt expressions of feelings and displays of emotion, and which promotes the traditional sex-role stereotyping and ideology of self-reliance, is also believed to be more pronounced in rural compared to urban communities (Komiti et al., 2006; Fuller, Edwards, Procter, & Moss, 2000). Seeing seeking help from professionals as a sign of personal weakness, over 80% of respondents in the study by Komiti and colleagues agreed that a person should work out their own problems while consulting professionals as a last resort and more males than females endorsed this. Good and Wood (1995) suggest that men's attitudes could be altered by reinterpreting psychological help-seeking as a behaviour requiring personal courage and strength, which would be consistent with traditional masculinity ideology.

Stigma of Mental Illness

See Impedance of Help-seeking and Impedance of Treatment and Recovery in Chapter 4

8 Help-Seeking Determinants and Instrumental Barriers

The Social Network

The social network has been referred to as a network of potential consultants (Angermeyer, Matschinger, & Riedel-Heller, 2001). It consists of multiple spheres of influence, each defined by its proximity to the individual, from the intimate and informal confines of the nuclear family through successively more select, distant, and authoritative laymen until the professional is possibly reached (Cauce et al., 2002; Rogler & Cortes, 1993). The intervention of the social network is a critical factor in help-seeking behaviour, especially in traditionalist communitarian systems (Barksdale & Molock, 2008). It influences the conceptualisation and interpretation of psychopathological symptoms, stereotypes regarding the effectiveness of given care pathways, coping mechanisms and the ultimate decision on which caregiver to consult (Sorketti, Zuraida, & Habil, 2013).

Cauce and colleagues (2002) illustrate the dynamics of the social network with the example of an African American mother of a seemingly depressed child who may consult her own mother, her sister, her best friend, and the family priest to get their opinions on whether her child's problem is serious or worthy of attention. Each conversation may alternately increase or decrease her level of worry and a corresponding commitment to seek help. If this round of consultation leads to a conviction to seek help, another round of consultation might ensue regarding what type of help that should be sought. In another example, a study that explored the perceived norms of mental health help-seeking among African American College Students found that family norms made a unique significant prediction of help-seeking intentions (Barksdale & Molock, 2008).

In communitarian cultures such as the Igbo of south-eastern Nigeria, the family forms the basic unit of the social network and is the customary starting point of the help-seeking pathway. The decision to seek help for mental or psychological problems, and the pathway to be explored, is a collaborative family effort which usually crystallises from a deliberative decision of the adult family members, with possible input from close associates including extended family members and friends. Relatives equally take it as their responsibility to prompt a member who demonstrates the need for help to seek help urgently.

While studies conducted in Western cultures cautiously noted that an attitude towards mental health services is 'partially' transmitted by family and friends (Angermeyer et al., 2001; Rickwood & Braithwaite, 1994), the decisive influence of the social network in collectivist cultures was exemplified in the finding that relatives initiated contact for the first treatment option in nearly 91% of cases in a study of an Igbo sample whereas only 9% was initiated by the patients themselves (Aniebue & Ekwueme, 2009). A study that investigated care-seeking of psychiatric patients in northern Nigeria found that for over four in five of patients, contact with the first healer was initiated by the patients' relatives with only 3% of first contacts being initiated by the patients themselves (Aghukwa, 2012).

Another study which investigated pathways to mental healthcare in northern Nigeria noted that sources of information about available mental health facilities came mostly from community members and neighbours (65%) ahead of the mass media (15%) (Abdulmalik & Sale, 2012). Hence, while social networking is only beginning to be encouraged in the West, for example, encouraging spouses to come to an initial appointment (Cusack, Deane, Wilson, & Ciarrochi, 2004), and calls are made for the creation of social advocacy groups that include partners, friends, family, and individuals from the community (Byrne, 2000), such practices are normative in collectivist cultures.

Cameron and colleagues (1993) found that 50% of those who sought medical services in the US were prompted to go by a significant other. They also found that 92% of those who sought medical care (as opposed to 61% of those who did not) talked to at least one person about their problem before seeking professional medical help. These corroborate the suggestion by Cauce and colleagues (2002) that social networks may have their greatest impact at the point of service selection in the help-seeking process because of their strong influence on real decisions about treatment.

It has been noted that, if the need to go for mental health assessment and treatment is strongly supported by the family, it does often work (Thornicroft, 2008), while living alone at the time of onset, and experiencing a lack of family involvement on the pathway to care increased the likelihood of a negative care pathway being taken (Anderson, Fuhrer, & Malla, 2010; Morgan et al., 2005). In developing collectivist cultures, the family cares for both the majority of clients who are outpatients due to a lack of admission facilities and those who are admitted in care. The latter is reinforced in Nigeria by a care policy whereby one close relative must stay with a patient on admission (Aniebue & Ekwueme, 2009).

Donnelly (1992) observed that a family-oriented psycho-educational approach was more effective in treating immigrants from collectivist cultures in an individualistic Western environment than an individual modality alone. Family collaboration is likely to increase the psychiatric clients' treatment adherence and follow-up in the community in these cultures. Hsu (2003) had indicated that a family-oriented psycho-educational approach could enlighten family caregivers in such areas as medication regimens, especially monitoring medication in order to prevent relapses.

Social networks can influence the help-seeking behaviour of people suffering from mental disorder, as a communication system by providing information and links, as a reference system by formulating normative expectations, and as a support system by providing care, reporting symptoms and helping patients cope with psychosocial stressors especially where the healthcare system is less developed (Angermeyer et al., 2001; Bergner et al., 2008; Wong, 2007a,b).

Boerner (2009) exemplified the importance of the traditional support of family friends with the story of Nancy Sharby, a mother of two children suffering from bipolar disorder in the US. She could not have her children treated because their insurance plan did not cover mental health since, as she lamented, "... the brain is the only organ in the body that requires its own insurance policy." Nancy had to fall back on a friends and family network support system. She confessed: "If I didn't know the people I know, I never would have gotten the services I did for my kids .... Both my kids have told me that if I didn't do what I did for them, they'd be dead or psychotic by now, because they were very, very sick. You can't advocate for yourself when you're psychotic. But even if you're not psychotic, you still can't fight for yourself if you don't know the system .... I have friends who are psychiatric nurses, social workers, insurance brokers, and if I didn't have all those pieces, I couldn't have gotten the services I did for my kids."

In a study by Dow and Woolley (2012), Albanian respondents described the close-knit nature of the family as the most important thing in life, and the main source of help and support for coping with various problems, including mental health issues. Family bonds and obligations were described as so strong that family members were reportedly willing to make sacrifices such as deciding not to get married or to quit jobs in order to care for sick loved ones. The family was described as the first, and sometimes the only place, for seeking help, especially with mental health problems. Family members would neglect their own mental health as they carried the burden of caring for one of their own with mental health problems.

In collectivist cultures, people do not distinguish their own interests from those of the group, and they perceive the self as intertwined and bound to others. While Western cultural values emphasise individualism, success, competition, and intellectualism – values that may inhibit Westerners from turning to the informal network for help for fear that it may be interpreted as a sign of weakness (Tzahr-Rubin, 2003), family and primary group relations are central and highly valued in collectivist cultures with their emphasis on the collective over the individual. This enables mutual aid and reliance on informal help over professional mental health facilities, which, from the perspective of the communitarian settings, have the potential to isolate the patient.

However, while the social network can provide care, and report symptoms, and could be an important source of advice and information for health-related issues, the complex dynamics of the social network could also mean that it might inhibit prompt seeking of mental healthcare. For instance, help from the social network (family, extended family, friends, and community members) in the communitarian societies is normally unsolicited – the goodwill of every community member in volunteering assistance is presumed, and every suggestion at the time of crisis, whether potentially helpful, harmful, or even contradictory is open to consideration and often favourably so. At times, rivalry can arise between the different arms of the network regarding whose opinion should hold sway, and this could add to the stress of the situation while also hampering decisive intervention.

The quality of the social network is also a factor; a social network with less mental health literacy could keep recycling ignorance to the detriment of the patient. It is noted that social networks delay in their recognition of the first signs of mental illness hence impeding prompt intervention and that families and friends most often suggest seeking care mostly when socially disturbing symptoms become prominent (Gater, Jordanova, Maric, & Alikaj, 2005; Mkize & Uys, 2004). Furthermore, as Mkize and Uys observed, with the structure of the family in the communitarian African system whereby there is usually the adult (male) head that takes the final decision on issues, there could be a delay in the decisive intervention in the event of a sudden crisis, in the absence of a family head in distant employment.

While limited social networks predicted restricted utilisation of mental health resources in one study (Bonin, Fournier, & Blais, 2007), research also hints at the irony of the inhibitive influence of tightly meshed social networks that could lead to delay in contacting health facilities (Rogler & Cortes, 1993; Lin, Inui, Kleinman, & Womack, 1982). When networks are open, and the individuals are not too involved with each other, they are more exposed to information about the environment, including where to go for professional treatment. People may be pressured towards the acceptance of normative beliefs that could run contrary to formal help-seeking in close-knit networks. The impact of the normative expectations could be felt in the finding that networks afraid of stigmatisation delay contact with psychiatric services (Angermeyer et al., 2001).

Moreover, collectivist cultures with strong community support systems and interlocking community and familial networks could also feel able to meet their needs from within; hence they will be reluctant to seek external help (Gilbert et al., 2007; Tata & Leong, 1994). Social conflicts arising from the closely knit and communal lifestyles of most African societies have also been associated with the emanation of distress (Asuni, Schoenberg, & Swift, 1994). Stigma and discrimination are particularly significant in collectivist societies where communities are smaller, social networks are closely enmeshed, and privacy is lacking (Barney, Griffiths, Jorm, & Christensen, 2006). Thus, social proximity can be a double-edged sword in the sense that, while the stronger sense of community may be a protective factor which offers higher social capital, the experience of social stigma may be more pronounced in such closely enmeshed communities.

Experience of the Mental Health System

Experience of mental health services is a significant determinant of future or continued service use (Gulliver, Griffiths, & Christensen, 2010; Kelly, Jorm, & Wright, 2007). Culturally, psychiatric treatment is a potentially difficult, embarrassing, and overall risky enterprise with respect to the individual's sense of self-worth and environmental homeostasis owing to the debilitating stigma surrounding mental illness. It may be assumed that by virtue of their training and dedication, health professionals are likely to have positive attitudes towards people with mental illness. However, this assumption does not always hold true as many studies have revealed a significant negative attitude of health workers towards mental illness (Hansson, Jorrnfeldt, Svedberg, & Svensson, 2013; van Boekel, Brouwers, van Weeghel, & Garretsen, 2013; Wahl & Aroesty-Cohen, 2010). Disturbingly, as Sartorius (2002) suggests, the stigma of mental illness begins with the attitudes and behaviour of medical professionals (iatrogenic stigma). This is most detrimental because of the belief that if a specialist says or thinks 'it is bad', then 'it is bad'. Negative experiences with mental health services can lead to mistrust of the system and the professionals, and these incidents are noted to inform reluctance to seek professional help (Howerton et al., 2007).

Ogborn (1995) recounts the many aspects of mental health treatment that give patients serious concern: regarding medication, they worry about the effectiveness, the side effects, and the risk of drug addiction; they feel concerned about the effectiveness and the frequency of the counselling or consultation sessions, the time necessary to complete the treatment; they are troubled that they must talk about private matters and sometimes painful experiences to others. Patients would, therefore expect that specialists are professional and empathetic: highly trained, educated, oriented to the problem, and interested in the personality of their clients and the clients' health status. However, these expectations may not always be confirmed in their experience.

Sartorius (2002) observed that psychiatrists have on occasions re-quested longer holidays and a higher salary than other doctors because they had to work with 'mentally ill patients who are dangerous'. They have also recommended separate legislation for people with mental illness 'to protect themselves' which can further set people with mental illness apart. Such arbitrary behaviours as unwillingness to offer services, overestimation of danger, excessive physical restrictions and over-sedation have been attributed to trained psychiatric personnel (Livaditis, 1994).

Read and Baker (1996) report that the most 'intolerant' group of employers were within health and social care, with the worst cases of overt displays of negative attitudes reportedly coming from the nursing and social work professions. Some reports indicate that professionals demonstrate more negative attitudes than the general public. For in-stance, data from the Viewpoint survey (Henderson et al., 2012) sug-gested that between 2008 and 2009, after the *Time to Change* social marketing campaign began in January 2009 in the UK, the overall level of discrimination dropped, accounted for by reduced discrimination from a number of sources, including friends, family, neighbours, employers, and education professionals, but there was no reduction in reports of dis-crimination from either mental or physical healthcare professionals. This corroborates the suggestion that medical staff held negative attitudes toward people with mental illness which were not moderated by educa-tional and clinical experience (Fabrega, 1995; Shao et al., 1997).

Health professionals were also less optimistic about treatment out-comes for mental illness than the general public (Hugo, 2001). They also held pessimistic attitudes regarding the integration of persons with mental illness into society (Moldovan, 2007) which may result in providing ser-vices that hinder, rather than facilitate, community integration. For ex-ample, in order to enable the acceptance of persons with mental illness by the community, a group of them were trained to conceal their mental illness and avoid situations which might result in rejection (Link, Mirotznik, & Cullen, 1991). A review of the outcomes of these inter-ventions showed that, instead of facilitating community adjustment, these strategies produced more self-stigma and discouragement.

The overwhelming majority of treatment for mental health difficulties is performed by General Practitioners (GPs) since over 90% of clients are managed in primary care, which is preferred by clients and their families because it allows easy access to services, facilitates early diagnosis of problems, and prompts interventions in a person-centred, non-stigmatising environment (Jenkins & Karno, 1992; Tylee, 1999). Yet, evidence suggests that not all practitioners wish to provide mental healthcare at their clinics, partly because of a lack of knowledge (King, Judd, & Grigg, 2001) but also because of a 'low therapeutic commitment' to this client group (Crawford & Brown, 2002). A community psychiatric nurse, in the study by Crawford and Brown, reports that '... there's still sort of a lot of stigma about mental health in GP surgeries ... they don't make the referrals at the appropriate time so we (mental health staff) tend to get them at crisis point, which can be disastrous .... You can really struggle to get through to the GPs as well.'

Some staff are unable to develop an essential rapport with mental health patients, and this can negatively affect outcomes for the patient (Friedman et al., 2005; Hawton, Daniels, & James, 1995). Psychiatrists rated mental health patients as 'difficult' 'annoying' and 'un-compliant' (Rao et al., 2009). Packer and colleagues (1994) found that medical residents believed they could not form a therapeutic alliance with patients suffering from chronic mental illness and would not be able to work with them in an individualised manner.

Fifty per cent of the nurses who participated in a study by Reed and Fitzgerald (2005) expressed a clear dislike of caring for people with mental health problems. Moreover, 27.6% of the doctors and 30.7% of the nurses in a study by Arvaniti and colleagues (2009) claimed that their job did not include services for persons with mental illness. Similar findings were reported by Björkman and colleagues (2008). A study of a Kenyan sample suggests that even if they were capable of handling psychiatric problems, general health workers preferred such patients to be managed by specialist mental health institutions to having them managed in general wards (Muga & Jenkins, 2008).

Health and social care professionals' attitudes and beliefs have a direct effect on the quality of care they provide (Griffiths & Pearson, 1988; Thornicroft, 2013) and can influence clinical outcomes of patients with mental illness (Schulze, 2007). Health workers may hold on to the mental illness stereotypes to treat the clients contemptuously. People with mental illness experience physical maltreatment in the hands of healthcare professionals and health workers, especially in general hospitals. These care providers also tend to favour isolation and custodial care of patients (Aghukwa, 2009a; Ewhrudjakpor, 2009).

Such negative approaches result in greater use of physical and chemical restraints on patients (Duxbury, 2002) which undermine their human rights (Hundertmark, 2002) and are objectionable to patients and relatives (Bonner, Lowe, Rawcliffe, & Wellman, 2002; Olofsson & Jacobsson, 2001). Observing a chronic psychiatric ward, Donati (2000) notes: "It seemed to me that, in response to the experience of failure and impotence in nursing chronic patients, there arises a defensive urge to extinguish any sign of spontaneity, involvement, emotionality and expectations, and to keep everything lifeless and predictable so as to avert new hopes, new disappointments and intensified frustration" (p. 41).

The negative experience of care can lead to treatment fearfulness – the subjective state of apprehension that arises from aversive expectations about the seeking and consumption of mental health services which is a leading barrier to help-seeking (Kushner & Sher, 1991; Zartaloudi & Madianos, 2010). Treatment fearfulness includes fear of embarrassment and change, fear of different stereotypes related to treatment, fear related to previous negative experiences of mental health services, and fear related to the treatment type. Negative experiences with psychiatric services may inhibit help-seeking when symptoms of a mental disorder first appear (Monteiro, Dos Santos, & Martin, 2006).

Forty-four per cent of people in London who had experienced mental distress reported having experienced discrimination from their GPs, while 35% reported experiencing discrimination from other health professionals (Rao et al., 2009). Service users have also indicated that some nursing staff in acute mental health settings do not display 'liking' towards them in terms of either friendly characteristics or behaviour (Hugo, 2001; The Mental Health Foundation of New Zealand, 2003).

Studies report that patients with mental illness feel that they are treated contemptuously and are made to wait longer than other patients. They often feel ignored, ridiculed or face the suspicion that their physical complaints may only be figments of their imagination. They experience a lack of interest in them and the history of their mental health problem. They reckon that health professionals are ignorant of the side effects of medication and that psychiatric diagnoses are mostly given with a negative prognosis (Liggins & Hatcher, 2005; Schulze & Angermeyer, 2003). Patients also express fear of breaches of confidentiality which could discourage them from seeking help from professionals (Corrigan, 2004).

Some Asian women express fears that confidentiality concerning any sensitive information about their mental states and difficulties, which they might share, including with their GP, may be compromised (Gilbert, Gilbert, & Sanghera, 2004). The insensitivity of professionals sometimes violates the implicit norms of good practice. A community health worker reports ' ... [A] woman ... was having regular visits from a Community Psychiatric Nurse who was female, and that wasn't a problem because it was like a friend going round. Then one day, a man actually turned up with a depot injection in his hand, so that everybody was looking out, and they could see the injection, so it was quite clear that there was something wrong, with ... suitcase, syringe in one hand, you know big nice [healthcare trust] badge, no sort of attempt to cover it up. And after that injection, she said well forget it, I'm not having any more injections, you know' (Crawford & Brown, 2002).

Psychiatric practice, in general, was found to generate exclusion and stigmatisation of persons with mental illness (Hugo, 2001). Sociological literature has suggested arguably that stigma has been thrust upon persons with mental illness by the psychiatric health system which could be seen as being concerned with containment, control, medication, or therapy while clients suffered stigma as a result of their often compulsory engagement with it (Crawford & Brown, 2002).

The social labelling processes discussed in Chapter 1 can be very salient in the mental health system, doing much damage. Labelling could be so thoroughly if unwittingly, integrated professionally and organisationally into the system (i.e. becoming part and parcel of the system) that removing it or even significantly diminishing its efficacy would have rocked the institution. Sartorius (2002) observed that the careless use of diagnostic labels is a major contribution by medical professionals to the stigmatisation of psychiatric disorders, and the World Health Organisation has identified this as a target for its campaign against stigma. Diagnostic terms can be useful in summarising information about a patient's illness and facilitate communication among professionals, but they can be harmful when used carelessly by professionals or when left at the disposal of non-professionals who are not familiar with the original definitions of the terms.

As gatekeepers of information and services, the opinion of mental health professionals, or their manner of presentation of mental illness and those who suffer from it, may greatly affect users' responses to professional intervention. The mental health workers' perception of their client's place in society also matters a great deal as it is likely to influence the client's motivation, compliance, and investment in the therapeutic relationship (Moldovan, 2007).

The potential adverse impact of negative attitudes of health workers is worse than the stigma maintained by the public in three ways. First, given that health workers usually have high social and intellectual status and are looked up to in their communities, their stigmatising attitudes can promote stronger public stigma through social modelling. Secondly, stigmatising attitudes of health workers can result directly in poor and suboptimal care for affected patients. Thirdly, as health workers are usually involved with the training of other workers and members of the public, their own prejudices and stereotypical views of mental illness could be transmitted with authority to their trainees making such views more likely to become internalised.

Surveys of medical staff in Nigeria showed that, despite their relatively impressive mental health literacy, they still harboured deeply rooted cultural beliefs that discriminated against those with mental illness resulting in their placing emphasis on custodial care and opposing care in the community (Aghukwa, 2009a; Ewhrudjakpor, 2009). Sixty-four per cent of medical doctors in selected health institutions in Nigeria preferred high social distance from people with mental illness (Adewuya & Oguntade, 2007). These were unwilling to share a room with someone with mental illness, which suggests an unwillingness to offer medical consultations that usually takes place in consulting rooms.

In the study by Aghukwa (2009a), almost two-thirds of medical staff (64.1%) would feel fearful at the thought of having people with mental problems admitted within the hospital, and more than half (53.0%) would not wish to have their place of work next door to the psychiatric wards. These corroborate the findings of the case study of south-eastern Nigeria

(Ikwuka, 2016) whereby 79.3% of the nurses would not want close association with people with mental illness while a third (35.4%) would be unwilling to relate with them even from a distance, and more than half (58.6%) would support authoritarian attitudes towards them which see them as different.

Furthermore, the association of mental illness with the abuse of substances in this region which has often provoked moralistic and stereotyping attitudes in health and social care professionals also result in punitive and rejecting responses, and interaction characterised by suspicion, mistrust and avoidance. Disturbingly, iatrogenic stigma persists in these contexts even in the absence of aberrant behaviour. This is exemplified by the findings of the aforementioned case study, whereby the negative responses of nurses prevailed even when the question on attitudes was in relation to people already cured of mental illness.

That health workers hold stigmatising attitudes despite their training and dedication to care may be explained by Modified Labelling Theory which suggests that such attitudes are learnt early in life through socialisation (Link, Cullen, Struening, Shrout, & Dohrenwend, 1989). The demanding nature of mental health services often generates anxiety amongst staff as they work under pressure which could lead to a form of 'misdirected aggression'. Health professionals also report poor knowledge and skills, lack of support, and the need for ongoing assistance and training to provide effective care (King et al., 2001; Muirhead & Tilley, 1995).

The General Nurses studied by Reed and Fitzgerald (2005) disliked and avoided caring for persons with mental illness because they were unsure of their responsibilities. However, they displayed positive attitudes when given support. Adequate support would bolster the confidence of healthcare providers which would likely animate the system and motivate the users too. Bailey (1998) reports that poor institutional support results in counter-productive coping tactics like tearoom humour as stress is released. Venting feelings this way could further perpetuate stereotypical negative responses.

Since persistence in the engagement process is the crucial element of the therapeutic process (Gournay, 1996), negative attitudes of professionals would be a major barrier to accessing mental healthcare and is therefore deserving of utmost attention by all the stakeholders. As Ogborn (1995) rightly observed, the therapeutic relationship between the patient and the mental health specialist is a crucial interface for the evolution and the outcome of the process of help-seeking. Interpersonal confidence is a necessary element in the therapist/patient relationship for the patient to freely relay painful and personal, private information about their life and health, disclosing personal emotions and thoughts, and accepting guidance through difficult life changes.

Inadequacy of Services

In the less industrialised developing world, biomedical mental health facilities are inadequate, under-equipped, and relatively inaccessible, requiring high transport costs (Edelman, Kudzma, & Mandle, 2014; García-Moreno, 2002; Lecrubier, 2005). These deter individuals, especially those with lower incomes, from accessing such services while availability and relative affordability add to the appeal of alternative care pathways (Campbell-Hall et al., 2010; Roberts, 2001; Tang, Sevigny, Mao, Jiang, & Cai, 2007). Accessibility of care was noted as the most significant predictor of attitudes towards seeking professional help for mental illness among ethnic minority groups (Fung & Wong, 2007). Indeed, for many in these contexts, traditional healers may be the only affordable and accessible form of healthcare.

A study on the treatment of psychiatric disorders in India noted that paucity of biomedical facilities for psychiatry leads about 80% of the population to depend on indigenous treatments consisting of Ayurvedic and Unani systems of medicine, religious treatments consisting of prayers, fasting, etc., and also various witchcraft practices and magical rituals (Lahariya, Singhai, Gupta, & Mishra, 2010). Nigeria generally has very poor mental health infrastructure with about 250 psychiatrists for 200 million people (Akinkuotu & Aworinde, 2019) which approximates to one psychiatrist to 800,000 people. More than half of the respondents (57.8%) in the case study of south-eastern Nigeria (Ikwuka, 2016) could be constrained by instrumental barriers from seeking help for mental illness.

The Primary Health Care (PHC) system forms the bedrock of Nigeria's health policy (Federal Ministry of Health, 1991). The system is based on the Alma Ata Declaration of 1978 in Kazakhstan under the auspices of the World Health Organisation and UNICEF (WHO, 1978). Primary care is envisioned to offer the first contact, provide a comprehensive, continuous, and coordinated services for persons with health conditions and also display the capacity for prompt referrals to a higher level of care (Gureje et al., 2015). The idea is to support the care of the most common diseases found in the community, irrespective of their complexity, using scientifically sound and appropriate technology and making this service universally accessible to individuals and families in the community through their full participation (Awojobi, 2011).

The PHC structure is made up of interdependent sections such as community health workers, non-governmental organisations (NGOs), nurses, support groups and members of the community in general, who work together to fulfil the functions necessary for meeting the health needs of the society as a whole. In line with the WHO directive, the Nigerian Federal Ministry of Health (FMOH) added mental health as the ninth component of the PHC in 1989, identifying this as the only realistic way that mental health services could reach the population (Federal

Ministry of Health, 1991). The perceived advantages of PHC include relative availability, affordability, but, most importantly, that patients from the community are treated by people they can relate to.

One of the early large-scale comprehensive evaluations of the Primary Health Care service delivery in the developing world was carried out by Primary Health Care Operations Research (PRICOR), a USAID-financed project between 1985 and 1992. It spanned 12 countries and uncovered severe deficiencies in the diagnosis, treatment, and counselling of patients as well as in the supervision of health workers (De Geyndt, 1995). Community satisfaction with primary health services was low, especially regarding the interpersonal skills of health centre staff. To improve healthcare, supposedly through better financing of the primary care system, user fees were introduced following the Bamako Initiative of 1987 (UNICEF, 1988). Consequently, cost and perceived low quality of care became some of the main reasons why people did not attend Primary Health Care services in cases of illness.

Moreover, lack of political will, poor leadership, and corruption were continually the banes of the Nigerian system, against the backdrop of a wider African continent bedevilled by crises: internal strife, political instability, malnutrition, communicable diseases, poor manpower, poverty etc. With basic necessities of life under threat, including other aspects of the health sector competing for attention, such as the "double epidemic" of high infant and maternal mortality rates, and the HIV epidemic, it comes as no surprise that mental health concerns have not been a priority for governments and policymakers in the African continent (Gureje & Alem, 2000; World Health Organization, 2001b).

This is reinforced by structural discrimination – institutional practices and policies that work to the disadvantage of minority groups, even in the absence of individual prejudice or discrimination (see Chapter 4, Structural Discrimination). While the WHO recommended 5% of the Gross Domestic Product (GDP) to be allocated for mental health, less than 3% of GDP is spent on health in Nigeria and of this less than 1% is allocated to mental healthcare. Consequently, many years after its introduction into the Primary Health Care (PHC), mental healthcare appears non-existent at this basic level of care and is scarcely existent at the secondary level (Lawani, 2008).

A recent study (Anyebe, Olisah, Garba, & Amedu, 2019) demonstrates that mental health services at the primary healthcare level remain critically inadequate especially in resource-poor and crisis-stricken communities. Of the 47 Primary Health Care centres in three states in Northern Nigeria selected for the study, none was providing any formal mental health services. There were only a few, uncoordinated, services in some centres, essentially provided by individual Primary Health Care service providers, and, in one case, a non-governmental organisation. The researchers concluded that, at best, mental health services at all Primary

Health Care centres, in all the Local Government Areas in all the states visited, were scarce, poorly, and haphazardly provided or completely absent in the vast majority of the centres.

The provision of care is thus limited from the source. And this is in spite of the escalating mental health needs due to urbanisation, breakdown of traditional family structures and political and economic instability. The resultant system of paying out-of-pocket, without insurance cover, means that many families find it hard to afford care for their loved ones, especially for chronic cases. This has resulted in 70% of Nigeria's approximately 200 million people lacking access to modern mental health services (Omigbodun, 2001) while an estimated one billion pounds is spent annually by politicians and the affluent on medical trips abroad (Fabiyi, 2013).

The consequences of this include: increased self-medication, patronage of alternative sources including private health facilities, drug vendors and traditional healers (Nsereko et al., 2011; Uzochukwu & Onwujekwe, 2004). Approximately 70% of mental health services in Nigeria are provided by religious and spiritual healers (Adewuya & Makanjuola, 2009). A study that investigated the barriers to the utilisation of Primary Health Care in Plateau State, north-central Nigeria, found high costs of drugs (29%), service charges (19%), easy access to traditional healers (39%) and difficulty in getting transport to a health facility (30%) as leading barriers (Katung, 2001).

Another study that investigated the burden of schizophrenia on rural and urban families in south-southern Nigeria showed that users experienced financial burdens in accessing mental healthcare, keeping follow-up appointments, and paying for treatment. This resulted in many being unable to sustain the treatment, and consequent relapse (Jack-Ide & Uys, 2013). A related study of caregivers' burdens, and psychotic patients' perception of social support in Nigeria, indicates that service users lacking any form of social welfare support had higher burdens, experienced more family dysfunction and poor illness outcomes (Ohaeri, 2001).

Murali and Oyebode (2004) observed how poverty could lead to maladaptive behaviours or the taking of questionable pathways, not with harmful intent, but as coping behaviours to provide comfort or relief from a stressful life. While drug peddlers, drug store operators, and traditional and faith healers may provide services that are closer to the people and may be cheaper in the short run than services from the biomedical healthcare providers (Asenso-Okyere et al., 1998), the adverse consequences of these measures include: over-dosing, problems of resistance, delay in arriving at standard medical facilities and discontinuing therapy (Awojobi, 2011; Deressa, Ali, & Enqusellassie, 2003; Gureje & Lasebikan, 2006; McCombie, 2002). Lacking access to effective mental healthcare results in the chronicity of mental illness with the attendant disease and stigma burdens. A study that examined attitudes toward people living with schizophrenia found that the public felt more positively towards sufferers who were in treatment than it felt about those that were not in treatment (NAMI as cited in Kobau, DiIorio, Chapman, & Delvecchio, 2010).

Reviews note lack of accessibility to healthcare facilities especially in rural populations (Fox, Blank, Rovnyak, & Barnett, 2001; Gulliver et al., 2010); rural people reported not knowing who to seek help from (Wrigley, Jackson, Judd, & Komiti, 2005). With policies that locate mental health institutions mainly in urban areas and big cities, the majority of Nigeria's population who live in poverty in rural areas lack access to modern mental health services due to poor knowledge of available services, the high cost of service including transport, and a negative view of the care system as elitist. Moreover, very few qualified practitioners would be ready to agree to work in rural areas where basic infrastructure, equipment and social amenities are lacking.

Thus, the majority of psychiatric presentations seen by clinicians are in primary care settings that are clearly not well equipped to be the main source of mental healthcare for people with severe mental disorders. In a South African study, staff in primary care lacked the skill to identify psychological distress, for instance, when clients presented physical symptomatology (Mkize & Uys, 2004). Another South African study reported significant problems of non-detection in primary care, whereby many with psychiatric disorders are either undiagnosed or misdiagnosed, resulting in inadequate treatment (Freeman, 1992). Lacking the skills translate to lacking in confidence; hence many of the primary care providers are basically not comfortable dealing with mental healthcare (Geller, 1999).

Primary Health Care workers in Africa themselves face many challenges that further inhibit their productivity, such as not receiving incentives for the work they do, the often uncooperative disposition of some community members including community leaders, and the lack of the basic tools of work such as transport to reach remote areas, which limits the spread of coverage. Lack of incentives could translate to a lack of commitment.

The PHC is designed to offer treatment and care in a continuum that is supported by a referral system (Obioha & Molale, 2011) but, in the Nigerian context, official referral procedures for referring persons from primary care to secondary/tertiary care and vice versa do not exist (WHO, 2011). There is also a lack of coordination of mental health services across the primary, secondary, and tertiary tiers of the health system with the result that needs do not determine the extent of the service provided. For example, a national survey found that a disproportionate number of persons with mild mental health conditions received specialist care while those with more severe conditions continued to receive inadequate care at the primary care level (Wang et al., 2007).

Lack of specialist mental healthcare in the system implies that communities would increasingly depend more on General Practitioners (GPs). Yet, a lot of factors can contribute to GPs not being in a position to provide optimal services. These include: lack of training and experience in psychiatry, absence of incentives, poor communications between the general practitioners and psychiatrists, regulations limiting the autonomy of general practitioners in managing mental disorders, and non-availability of medication (Gater, Jordanova, Maric, & Alikaj, 2005). GPs' low therapeutic commitment to this client group could also be informed by the stigmatised image of the mental patient and the myth of incurability.

Ultimately, therefore, psychiatric facilities in Nigeria are basically limited to tertiary institutions. Yet, provision of care at this level is also undermined by systemic, infrastructural, and logistical constraints. For instance, unevenly scattered around Nigeria, a country of about 200 million people, are 31 psychiatric facilities, all situated in urban areas and virtually having no synergy with health facilities in the community such as the district general hospital in each Local Government Area and the four to seven PHC centres within a Local Government Area, each of which serves 10,000 to 30,000 people (Omigbodun, 2001). These limited under-equipped mental health institutions are riddled with and disrupted by persistent staff strike actions that encourage the 'brain drain' which is evident in the migration of professionals, with the result that there are more Nigerian psychiatrists in Britain alone than in Nigeria (Ewhrudjakpor, 2010b).

A report (Njoku, 2015) described one of the Neuropsychiatric Hospitals as a battlefield with a lingering crisis between the management and workers concerning the conditions of service. This has crippled operations, resulting in the main entrance to the hospital being under lock and key for years, and the hospital premises being described as "home to uncompleted and abandoned projects, with inadequate wards to accommodate referred patients." Also reported was the non-availability of work materials such as reagents for the laboratories and drugs for pharmacies resulting in patients resorting to roadside pharmacies for prescriptions. Prohibitive user fees also contribute to the diminishing access to care in these tertiary health institutions (Awojobi, 2011). Moreover, the practice of public doctors running private clinics alongside their public role potentially compromises the system, with the possibility of doctors having divided loyalties and a situation whereby the doctors could exploit public facilities as feeder systems for their private practices.

Case for Integrated Primary Care

The Primary Health Care (PHC) initiative is meant to decentralise healthcare down to community level, but the absence of effective community-based mental health services puts additional pressure on the already stretched tertiary facilities. Moreover, the logistics of accessing tertiary-based care in urban centres can cost more for people from rural communities. Having to trek or travel long distances to access care entails taking time away from trade, work, or home responsibilities. In a study of south-southern Nigeria (Jack-Ide, Uys, & Middleton, 2013), the distance travelled to access service was of great concern resulting in many families not sustaining or continuing with treatment.

It has been shown that those living closer to services demonstrate shorter delays in arriving at services (Gater et al., 1991), which suggests that decentralising psychiatric services and providing local access might diminish delays. Furthermore, given that initial recognition and response to mental health problems generally takes place in the community (Angermeyer et al., 2001), there is need for the integration of quality mental health services into Primary Health Care as a way of facilitating early detection and intervention for mental disorders, in keeping with the ideals of the Alma-Ata declaration that inspired the Primary Health Care model.

The World Health Organisation (WHO) (2008) makes the case that effectively integrating mental health services into primary care is the most viable way of closing the treatment gap and ensuring that people get the mental healthcare they need. Since mental and physical health problems are interwoven, and many people suffer from both physical and mental health problems, integrated primary care services would help to ensure that people are treated in a holistic manner – meeting the mental health needs of people with physical disorders, as well as the physical health needs of people with mental disorders.

With such a model, patients would be handled by staff who know their cultural background and context, which would forestall some of the therapeutic dissonances that usually arise when patients are treated outside their socio-cultural milieu, by people who may not be familiar with the culture and the situation in which the patients live. An integrated model would also support people to access mental health services in close proximity to their homes which would help to keep families together – an ideal in communitarian societies.

Primary care for mental health would also facilitate community outreach and mental health promotion, as well as long term monitoring and management of affected individuals. Mental health services delivered in primary care holds more promise for the minimisation of stigma and discrimination as the effects of institutional treatment would be forestalled. Trained PHC staff can provide preventive interventions that do not necessarily need a high level of expertise; hence the model would make for a generally cost-effective care system by curbing the wasteful deployment of highly specialised professionals who may end up treating milder forms of illness that could be handled very well by practitioners at primary care centres.

Disturbingly, the attitude of Primary Health Care workers is one barrier to the integration of mental health services into Primary Health Care. A cross-sectional survey of south-western Nigeria using the Community Attitudes towards Mental Illness (CAMI) scale showed that primary care workers had attitudes similar to those seen in the general population (Mosaku & Wallymahmed, 2017). Another study of Primary Health Care workers in south-western Nigeria (Ogunlesi & Adelekan, 1988) suggests that general awareness of mental health principles is low. Nine in ten of the respondents believed that mental disorders might have a supernatural basis and half of the respondents believe that mental illness is transmissible through breastfeeding.

Only one out of every ten respondents had previously had to deal with patients with mental illness at their centres, an indication that the generality of the people at the grassroots level in the local government area were yet to identify mental health services within the Primary Health Care facilities. Similarly, half of the respondents reported that their centres were unable to offer any emergency treatment to an acutely disturbed patient. More significantly, about half of the care workers did not go through mental health education during their training. These formed the bulk of those who believed that mental disorder could be transmitted by a bite from a lunatic. The majority of the respondents that preferred not to attend to patients with mental illness at their health centres also came from this group.

Integration of mental health services in primary care needs a system of education and enlightenment to succeed. The WHO (2008) recognised that certain skills and competencies are required to effectively assess, diagnose, treat, support, and refer people with mental disorders and that primary care workers must be adequately equipped with these skills and competences. From an international study of mental health patients presenting in PHC services in developing countries, it was demonstrated that it is possible to train general and PHC staff in methods of treatment of several mental disorders, and that staff so trained can provide useful and effective services to clients (Gater et al., 1991).

Evidence now abounds, also from the Nigerian context, that Primary Health Care workers can be trained in skills that would enable them to deliver both psychological and pharmacological treatments. Gureje and colleagues (2015) successfully conducted a pilot programme to integrate mental health services into primary healthcare in Nigeria using the WHO Mental Health Gap Action Programme Intervention Guide (mhGAP-IG), contextualised for the local setting. The programme was implemented over 18 months in eight selected Local Government Areas (LGAs) in Osun state, south-western Nigeria. A well-supervised cascade training model was utilised for the programme with Master Trainers providing training for the Facilitators, who, in turn, conducted several rounds of training for frontline Primary Health Care workers. A total of 198 primary care workers, from 68 primary care clinics, drawn from eight Local Government Areas with a combined population of 966,714, were trained in the detection and management of mental, neurological and substance use (MNS) disorders, including moderate to severe major depression, psychosis, epilepsy, and alcohol use disorders. The study reported a marked improvement in the knowledge and skills of the health workers following training, and also a significant increase in the numbers of persons identified and treated for MNS disorders, and in the number of referrals.

It needs to be recognised, though, that inadequately trained PHC staff that are lacking especially in referral skills could do more harm than good in the care process. For instance, Fujisawa and colleagues (2008) discovered that, ironically, mental health professionals other than psychiatrists, who were consulted prior to accessing psychiatric care, delayed patients' referral to the psychiatric system more often than the non-healthcare professionals such as social workers. This somewhat reflects the local saying that 'Half education is dangerous.' Perhaps, armed with their limited knowledge, the mental health professionals were tempted to push their luck with the patients instead of making prompt referrals, while those lacking in any knowledge, and recognising their limitations, promptly referred patients to the specialists. PHC staff need, therefore to learn referral skills, which they need to apply promptly as part of professional competence.

The WHO further notes that integration is most successful when mental health is incorporated into health policy and legislative frameworks and is supported by senior leadership, adequate resources, and ongoing governance. It is therefore important that governments at the federal and local levels demonstrate political will and commitment to the policy through adequate financing and provision of opportunities for training of staff, including scholarship schemes. To succeed, integration of mental health services into primary care also needs to be accompanied by complementary services, particularly secondary care components, to which primary care workers can turn for referrals, support, and supervision.

It is thus a disturbing observation (Sartorius, 1998) that psychiatrists who are in a position to foster these integrated services feel threatened that their jobs might be usurped, and their income diminished with the integration of mental healthcare into PHC, and the involvement of GPs. This leads to the reluctance of many towards the integration model and the delegation of mental health tasks to general healthcare workers. The psychiatrists, therefore, constitute an important demographic for targeted advocacy necessary to sensitise stakeholders, including national and local political leadership, health authorities, management, and primary care workers, to the overall gains of such a cost-effective model of mental healthcare. This is especially considering the prevalence of mental disorders, the burden they impose if left untreated, the human rights violations that often occur in psychiatric hospitals and the positive impact of well managed primary care-based treatments. Ultimately, the ideal of a complementary model of care (see Chapter 12), whereby the alternative care providers could work alongside biomedical practitioners, is most feasible with the primary care model which is designed to operate at the basic social structure as the alternative models.

However, the call to integrate mental healthcare into primary care is not without some concerns. It has been feared that integration may impose Western medical treatment models, undermine other healthcare sectors such as the district or secondary tier levels and could result in a failure to address and strengthen community rehabilitation (Sartorius, 2014; Ventevogel, 2014). Experience from other sub-Saharan African countries has also raised concerns about poor policy implementation, shortage of health professionals to drive and support the process, poor community engagement and mobilisation, and lack of medications (Bhana, Petersen, Baillie, & Flisher, 2010; Petersen, Ssebunnya, Bhana, & Baillie, 2011).

9 Ideological vs. Instrumental Barriers

Contrary to expectation, the case study of south-eastern Nigeria (Ikwuka, 2016) found that ideological barriers were perceived significantly more (83.3%) than instrumental barriers (57.8%). This indicates that inadequacy of services and material poverty, which are easily perceived as the major barriers to good mental healthcare in the developing world, may, after all, not be as inhibitive as socio-cultural factors, stigma and shame, cultural (in)appropriateness of care, the conceptualisation of mental illness, mental health literacy, and a culture of self-reliance. The finding has crucial policy implications. It suggests the likelihood of services being underused even if improved, which corroborates the disturbing observation that most people with psychological distress receive no mental health treatment even when care is free.

Thus, it demonstrates that determining the conceptualisation of mental illness could help in unravelling the reasons for the underutilisation of mental health services. A key policy implication here is the need to prioritise mental health education and cultural competency in care for optimal service uptake. However, the study also revealed a strong positive relationship between perceived ideological and instrumental barriers which reflects a link between ideological and material poverty. This, in consequence, corroborates the suggestion of the human capital theory (Tilak, 2002) which envisages a strong linear relationship between learning and earning, thus underscoring the interaction of ideological and instrumental factors in shaping help-seeking behaviour (Barker, Olukoya, & Aggleton, 2005).

Barriers to Help-Seeking: Socio-demographic Correlates

The World Psychiatric Association (WPA) underlines the necessity of selecting a target group when implementing educational activities and that a more specific definition of the target group facilitates the assessment of programme efficacy (WPA, 2005). The case study of south-eastern Nigeria found that the UK-based respondents would be potentially less constrained ideologically and instrumentally from seeking mental healthcare compared to the home- (Nigeria) based respondents. This is to be expected given the potential effects of acculturation and the more developed and accessible UK healthcare system. Barimah and Teijlingen (2008) did observe that culturally based behaviours change over time towards those prevalent in the host culture.

Yet, that as many as almost two-thirds (63.9%) of the sample could still be inhibited by ideological barriers is indicative of the fact that acculturation might not be enough to prompt an immigrant population in a host Western culture to robustly pursue mental care. Moreover, besides the fact that acculturation itself demands changes in orientation which may engender its own conflicts, studies have shown that higher orientation towards the host culture has not always been found to be an indicator of positive outcomes among immigrants. For instance, Clark and Hofsess (1998) found that an increased level of acculturation towards the host culture was associated with higher rates of depression, drug use, and mortality. A marginalised style of acculturation has also been associated with symptoms such as anxiety and depression (Neto, 2002).

On the other hand, immigrants who identified with their native cultures were found to have more favourable psychological adjustment, and this is after controlling for personality and self-efficacy differences (Chen, Benet-Martinez, & Bond, 2008). This shows that, notwithstanding the prospects of acculturation, immigrants' autonomy should not be significantly compromised as they contend with the systems of the host culture, which need to demonstrate sensitivity. It has been observed that health professionals' lack of cultural competency, including adequate knowledge and awareness of the impact of cultural differences in the assessment and treatment of mental illness, constitute additional barriers to the adequate accessing of mental healthcare by immigrants (Gaines, 1998; Idemudia, 2004).

The cultural understanding, meanings and symbols immigrants bring with them are critical in addressing immigrants' experiences. These were accentuated in the aforementioned critical study by Keynejad (2008), which explored the barriers that constrain ethnic minority groups from adequately accessing mental healthcare in London. Ethnic minorities in the study saw psychotic symptoms as spiritual and identified faith leaders as the appropriate persons to seek help from. They were quite suspicious of mental health services and were unconvinced that medication would be of any use. Many felt their problems to be social rather than medical, while others did not feel that primary care workers had any expertise in mental health. The study further identified that gossip, negative stereotypes, social rejection, and lack of understanding all made it harder for people to identify symptoms as a problem.

Moreover, many were unaware of the available help which could explain the finding of the case study (Ikwuka, 2016) that over a third (38.9%) of the UK-based Nigerian respondents could be constrained by instrumental barriers from accessing healthcare even in a relatively well-developed healthcare system. Keynejad (2008) also reported that those who did access services sometimes found them to be far better than they had anticipated, which shows that people with limited information may overestimate their reservations. Furthermore, the study reported that there was mistrust of the mental health system as people said they expected primary care practitioners not to have enough time to listen to them, to prescribe anti-depressants as a default solution, or be dismissive of their complaints. Users in the study felt their views were rarely consulted, yet many were not equipped with the procedures for registering their complaints should they feel dissatisfied with the services. Studies indicate that the experience or anticipation of unfair and unequal treatment in mental health services generates deeply entrenched mistrust within minority communities and acts as a powerful barrier to accessing care and treatment (Edge & Rogers, 2005; Keating, 2007; Keating, Bobertson, McCulloch, & Francis, 2002).

As a way forward, the respondents in the study by Keynejad (2008) wanted services to be delivered more holistically in the form of a complementary model with alternative therapies. Those not using the services wanted more information about the help available in their own languages, while those using the services wanted more information about their medication and treatment made available in their own languages. Following the study, the author suggested some steps with the potential to improve ethnic minorities' perceptions of mental health and help-seeking behaviour. These included:

1   Education and promotion that aim at myth-busting and raising the profile and accessibility of primary care
2   Provision of holistic healthcare such as low-intensity talking therapies delivered by ethnically diverse therapists
3   Greater involvement of ethnic minority service users in service user committees as well as one-off events, to consult service users and carers from specific ethnic minority communities in service planning and design
4   Establishment of a system that investigates ethnic minority carers' needs and determines gaps in the service
5   Cultural competence training delivered to a group of ethnically diverse service providers and clinicians, and provision of chaplaincy services across the diversity of ethnic groups and the breadth of faiths
6   Development of polyclinics which take on board the suggestions of service users towards the development of an integrated model that would incorporate faith, physical and mental health services

Although still somewhat contentious, the UK National Health Service (NHS) does currently provide some of the alternative therapies which may be a crucial way of engaging ethnic minority groups by illustrating that services go beyond the Eurocentric biomedical model. Though national interest in the mental health of ethnic minorities seems to have increased in the past decade, the human service professions have historically failed to meet the particular mental health needs of various underserved ethnic groups (Baruth & Manning, 2003). It is of particular concern that empirical investigations of mental health issues pertaining to Africans continue to lag behind in comparison to the volume of research conducted on other minority groups (Betancourt, Green, & Carrillo, 2000). The non-adaptation of services to the needs of African immigrants, and their unique struggles in adapting to a new culture and belief system, impose additional barriers for those of them that suffer from mental illnesses and need treatment.

Nurses in the case study (Ikwuka, 2016) demonstrated significantly less perceived ideological and instrumental barriers compared to the non-nursing occupational groups (students, teachers, and the general public). This would be expected given the training and experience of nurses that should help them burst myths surrounding mental illness, on the one hand, and also give them an advantage in terms of the pragmatics of accessing care. This furthermore underscores the importance of improving mental health literacy as key to emancipating people from ideological barriers that could inhibit them from promptly seeking mental healthcare.

However, the study showed that students significantly predicted perceived ideological barriers. This is disturbing, especially as the onset of serious mental illnesses like schizophrenia is mostly during adolescence and young adulthood (Kleintjes, Lund, & Flisher, 2010). It agrees with the consistent research finding that the gap in help-seeking for mental illness is most striking in young people (Rickwood, Deane, & Wilson, 2007; SAMHSA, 2012; Zachrisson, Rodje, & Mykletun, 2006). A systematic review of literature (Gulliver, Griffiths, & Christensen, 2010) also confirms the leading barriers to young people's access to mental health services are mostly ideological: stigma, embarrassment, lack of emotional competence and mental health literacy, concern with confidentiality and trust, and resort to self-help. Young adults also demonstrate more pessimism about treatment and prognosis (Kobau, DiIorio, Chapman, & Delvecchio, 2010). It is to be expected that the embarrassment and social isolation that come with stigma will be of exceptional concern for the young student in an age bracket that prizes social and peer acceptance, hence the reluctance to self-disclose, obsession with confidentiality, and recourse to self-help.

Secondly, as youth is stereotyped with anti-social behaviours, there is the likelihood that a society which causally links mental illness to substance abuse and moral failings could be quick to deplore the mental illness of the young as a product of self-destructive behaviour. This could discourage young people from disclosing mental health challenges as a system of adult providers would not earn their confidence. It could also explain why young people show greater help-seeking intentions towards trusted sources such as friends who share common experiences with them (Barker, Olukoya, & Aggleton, 2005; Rickwood, Deane, & Wilson, 2007). It was observed, however, that young people who have established relationships with health professionals were likely to seek help in the future (Rickwood, Deane, Wilson, & Ciarrochi, 2005). Interpersonal confidence is a necessary ingredient of therapy, particularly for the wary youth, to freely relay painful and personal information about their life and health, and to accept guidance through difficult life changes.

The failure to elicit the views of young people on the subject of mental health has been well documented (Department of Health [DOH], 2005; Parish, 2004). Disturbingly too, the review by Gulliver and colleagues (2010) also found that there is a paucity of high-quality research in the area of help-seeking determinants for young people. As an age bracket with a high risk of the onset of serious mental illness, this group would benefit from targeted interventions. Since stigma reduction during the adolescent years increases adolescents' comfort in discussing mental disorders (Pinto-Foltz & Logsdon, 2009), mental health education (which helps to normalise mental illness thereby reducing stigma) would be a promising intervention. Following an educational intervention in a research study, young people believed that people with mental illness were less distinct, less of a threat and less shameful, and there was no need to keep such people at a safe distance, restrict their activities or hide their mental illness (Pitre, Stewart, Adams, Bedard, & Landry, 2007). The school has proved to be an enabling platform for health promotion schemes (Gale, 2001; Lauria-Horner, Kutcher, & Brooks, 2004; Pinfold et al., 2003; Randhawa & Stein, 2007). Given the necessity of intervention at this stage, radical measures such as the inclusion of mental health literacy in the school curriculum could be decisive. Interventions in schools which facilitate encounters between students and people with schizophrenia have also proved to be particularly promising (Schulze, Richter-Werling, Matschinger, & Angermeyer, 2003; see also Chapter 6, Contact Theory).

Teachers in the case study (Ikwuka, 2016) also significantly predicted perceived ideological barriers which is disturbing, given that they should be instrumental in the improvement of mental health literacy through the school system. This is all the more worrying as it suggests the possibility that ignorance regarding mental illness is being recycled in the school system. It is therefore imperative that teachers are targeted for mental health education, not only for their own mental healthcare (which is crucial given their vulnerability in doing one of the most taxing but least remunerated jobs in the region) but also because of the ideological influence they wield over pupils, including those with mental illness.

The case study equally found that females could be more constrained by ideological barriers than males in seeking mental healthcare. This appears incongruent with the finding that females appear comparatively more positive towards mental illness (cf. Chapter 5, Demographic Correlates of Stigmatising Attitudes) and are also generally more favourably disposed towards seeking mental healthcare than males (Judd, Komiti, & Jackson, 2008; Mackenzie, Gekoski, & Knox, 2006; ten Have et al., 2010). However, besides the fact that females demonstrated more supernatural attribution for mental illness in an earlier study of the region (Ikwuka, Galbraith, & Nyatanga, 2014) which undermines the effectiveness of biomedical psychiatry and is consequently associated with less compliance with the biomedical treatment model (Kurihara, Kato, Reverger, & Tirta, 2006; Rose, 2010), a gender effect appears to be culturally mediated.

Studies that associate females with a greater disposition to seeking mental healthcare are mostly with Western samples. Most of the studies from the more traditionalist and collectivist developing world including Nigeria, report otherwise (Aniebue & Ekwueme, 2009; Gilbert et al., 2007; Lahariya, Singhai, Gupta, & Mishra, 2010). This might be attributed to the prevailing gender bias in these societies. For instance, help-seeking could cause potential damage to females' marital prospects in these cultures with the likelihood of divorce or husbands taking on second, polygamous wives (see Chapter 7, Culture). While a male marked as 'mentally ill' could easily contract marriage in most of sub-Saharan Africa, marriage is almost effectively foreclosed for a woman similarly identified.

The gender bias is further revealed in men and women, placing differential emphasis on the importance of the beliefs and values of their social networks. Whereas women who sought help were more likely to report that family members would not get upset on learning about it, there was no relationship between men's beliefs about family members' opinions and their use of therapy (Leaf, Livingston, & Tischler, 1986). Taking cognisance of gender differences in mental health, including risk and help-seeking, would ensure a more gender-sensitive approach in mental health policies.

The case study (Ikwuka, 2016) also found that low education significantly predicted perceived instrumental barriers. Access to information is vital for awareness and access of available services, and those with more education, invariably having better access to information, demonstrate higher rates of help-seeking and treatment utilisation (Al-Rowaie, 2005). In a typical south-eastern Nigeria village setting, information is disseminated to the people through limited channels such as church gatherings, town criers and mobile public address systems. The more educated people who can read, and who also have a better grasp of English, the official medium of communication, have wider access to information including from the print and electronic media.

People with limited information on the available biomedical mental health services may overestimate their inaccessibility. Furthermore, in keeping with the human capital theory, those with low education are also more likely to lack the material resources to access services. With a very low Tertiary Gross Enrolment ratio of 10% (UNESCO Institute for Statistics, 2011), the majority of Nigerians (90%) in the lower education category are therefore at risk of being impeded by instrumental barriers from accessing mental healthcare. This justifies the recommendation by the WHO to scale up mental health services in low and medium-income countries (WHO, 2010). This will involve making services available to more people who need them, increasing the range and variety of services offered, ensuring that services are culturally appropriate or well adapted to contexts and sustaining these services through effective policy, implementation, and financing.

Part III

Pathways to Mental Healthcare

Evolving an Effective Design

Introduction

Participation in the social system is always potentially relevant to the state of illness, to its aetiology and the conditions for successful therapy (Parsons, 1951). Thus, illness behaviour is a culturally and socially learned response to the extent that symptoms of any illness are differentially perceived, evaluated, and acted upon. Healthcare seeking behaviour is conceptualised as a sequence of remedial actions taken to rectify perceived ill-health (Ahmed, Adams, Chowdhury, & Bhuiya, 2000).

Pathways to mental healthcare are not random. While clinical factors such as symptom severity provide the impetus to the pathway, the decision to seek help, and the selection of a help provider are structured by the convergence of personal, developmental, psychosocial, cultural, systemic, and socio-economic factors (Cauce et al., 2002; Rogler & Cortes, 1993). These are reflected in the visibility or perceptual salience of the signs and symptoms, the extent to which the symptoms are perceived as serious, the degree that the symptoms disrupt family and social activities, the frequency and persistence of symptoms, and the tolerance threshold of the person experiencing the symptoms. They are also demonstrated in the available information and cultural assumptions of the person concerned, needs competing with illness responses, competing possible interpretations as to the causation of the symptoms, availability of treatment resources, physical proximity and the costs of treatment (Mechanic, 1968).

From a cognitive theory framework (Liang, Goodman, Tummala-Narra, & Weintraub, 2005), three identifiable stages characterise the help-seeking pathway: defining the problem, deciding whether to seek help, and finding a source of support. The first line of care experienced by person(s) with mental illness constitutes the most important stage of the psychiatric care pathway as delays in the initiation of appropriate treatment are associated with worse clinical and social outcomes including the exacerbation of symptoms, poor response to treatment, and poor quality of life (Adeosun, Adegbohun, Adewumi, & Jeje, 2013). Pathways to mental healthcare highlight popular beliefs about mental illness, the nature of accessible services and the choices that may have critical implications for the eventual outcome. An inclusive view of pathways to mental healthcare, with a complete mapping of care providers in the community, is necessary for the planning of mental health services and the evolution of a model of care that would respond more effectively to the cultural characteristics and contextual peculiarities of users.

10 Pathways to Mental Healthcare

The Biomedical Model

The typical biomedical model, characteristic of Western psychiatry, is dominated by the biomedical explanation for mental illness, with its emphasis on the diagnosis of symptoms which are treated primarily through medical interventions. In this model, General Practitioners (GPs) act as gatekeepers to psychiatric services, though a report indicated that the referral source for the greatest proportion of patients in this system is emergency services (Anderson, Fuhrer, & Malla, 2010). A deregulated form of this model, where patients can see any healthcare professional of their choice, with the possibility of having direct access to mental health professionals, is also available in some parts of the world such as Japan (Fujisawa et al., 2008) and Eastern Europe (Gater, Jordanova, Maric, & Alikaj, 2005). Direct access to mental health professionals makes for timely intervention, thereby shortening the duration of untreated illness, especially in cases with the potential to escalate beyond GPs' resolution. However, it could equally undermine the important gate-keeping roles of GPs who filter the care pathway, thereby ensuring a more cost-effective deployment of specialist services.

The 'Free Market' Model

Alternative (Faith/Spiritual and Traditional) healers play important roles alongside biomedical professionals in the 'free market' model found in the developing world, including sub-Saharan Africa. Often, a network of personal contacts is exhausted in this model before contact is made with professional services. The consideration of a variety of treatment options in this model aligns with the multiple and sometimes 'conflicting' beliefs that are held as potential causes of illnesses, as earlier noted. This 'cognitive tolerance' (MacLachlan, 1997) is reinforced by the holistic conception of human beings, with the health and well-being of people attributable to immediate or distant social, spiritual, and natural factors (Aghukwa, 2012; Westerlund, 1989).

Alternative institutional care in sub-Saharan Africa could be categorised into two types: syncretic religious (spiritual or faith) healers and traditional native doctors. While there are significant peculiarities, the two models often share a common recourse to the supernatural for both diagnosis and healing. Both often confirm the beliefs of patients, and diagnoses are normally tailored to meet the expectations of the clientele (Edwards et al., 1983; Sorsdahl et al., 2009). There is also a common tendency to mystify therapeutic procedures which work to inspire awe in clients and dispose them more confidently towards the therapeutic process (see *anwansi* and more in Chapter 7, Cultural (In)appropriateness of Care).

Spiritual Pathway (Faith Healers)

Faith healers in most of sub-Saharan Africa belonged to the African Initiated Churches (AIC) though many have sprung up from the mainline Catholic and Protestant churches. They adopt Christian, or integration of Christian and traditional healing methods, which include religious rituals such as: prayers, fasting, prophesying, exorcism, deliverance sessions, use of sacramentals (holy water, holy oils, burning of incense etc.), the offering of sacrifices, and the syncretic use of herbal and other concoctions (Lawani, 2008; Oyegbile, 2009). The treatment process could involve counselling but also confinement, flogging, chaining, and home visitation of patients to help them get rid of certain diabolical items which the healer claims had been used to bewitch the patient.

Faith healers use *anwansi* to earn the confidence of their clients, thus disposing them positively towards the therapeutic process. However, *anwansi* could also be manipulative – exploited to achieve selfish influence over gullible clients even if it entails using 'spiritual' blackmail on them. For instance, a pastor could prophesy impending doom or fortune over the client, which only he or she (the pastor) could forestall or mediate as applicable. In this way, such pastors secure their trade which thrives on their followers having perpetual recourse to them while they exploit them materially even at the risk of worsening clients' condition and possible death. In his play, *The Trials of Brother Jero*, which mirrors *The Pardoner's Tale* by Geoffrey Chaucer, the Nigerian Nobel Laureate for Literature, Wole Soyinka, illustrated this scenario. The dubious Prophet Jero deploys his mastery of manipulation to keep his followers subservient because he understands what they long for – wellbeing: money, social status, health, and power, and he convinces them that they will soon be able to fulfil these desires. His followers are gullible enough to believe him.

On the other hand, some faith healers in the region also provide social and material support for the usually destitute sufferers of serious mental illness. They place themselves at the meeting point between what they refer to as the backward and outdated traditional healers and the modern, scientifically based Western medicine (Freeman & Motsei, 1992). The significance of their service in the region is immediately evident, for instance, in over 90% of the population in south-eastern Nigeria being practising Christians for whom their faith is a way of life (Agbodike, 2008). Moreover, studies have considered the "spiritual" in users' experiences, which has helped to transform experiences positively (Clarke, 2001; Mental Health Foundation, 2002). The significance of the religious and spiritual experiences of users in offering comfort and support for mental health problems and during treatment in mental health institutions has also been acknowledged (Fallot, 2001; Harrison et al. 2001).

Traditional Pathway 1

Traditional medicine is the sum total of knowledge, skills and practices based on the theories, beliefs, and experiences indigenous to different cultures, whether explicable or not, used in the maintenance of health as well as in the prevention, diagnosis, improvement, or treatment of physical and mental illnesses (World Health Organization, 2002). Traditional healing practices could also involve medical and non-medical procedures including complex rituals such as: divination, the offering of supplications or sacrifices to appease the gods or ancestors (who could have inflicted the affliction), exorcism, use of charms and incantations (to ward off evil spirits), herbal medications and concoctions (Odejide, Oyewunmi, & Ohaeri, 1989). The treatment procedure could also entail confinement, flogging, chaining, and counselling.

Traditional healers utter incantations to potentiate medicines which are regarded as possessing their own "life force" and not just the chemical activity of constituent substances (Nwokocha, 2010). Diviners claim access to the supernatural realm, which enables them to unravel the cause of illness and misfortune. Hence, while laboratory services may be required to inform diagnosis and treatment in biomedical care, clients consult traditional healers for both causal explanations and the cure of their illness. *Anwansi* is the stock in trade of traditional healers who often anticipate and confirm the beliefs of patients. Diagnoses are normally tailored to meet the expectations of the clients. The popularity of traditional healers is further reinforced by their relative availability, accessibility, and affordability.

Traditional Pathway 2: The Social Network

(see Chapter 8)

11 Patterns of Mental Healthcare Pathways in Sub-Saharan Africa

A meta-analysis of studies investigating pathways to mental healthcare indicates an approximately equal initial choice of biomedical (49.2%) and alternative (48.1%) mental healthcare pathways in sub-Saharan Africa (Burns & Tomita, 2015). However, regional variations could also be observed. For instance, while studies from West and Eastern Africa report that more than half of patients initially took the alternative care pathways before arriving at biomedical psychiatric facilities, the reverse appears to be the case in southern Africa.

A study of south-western Nigeria found that about 70% of patients were treated by spiritual healers and 43% by traditional healers before presenting at a biomedical psychiatric facility (Agara & Makanjuola, 2006). In a later study of the same region (Adeosun, Adegbohun, Adewumi, & Jeje, 2013), patients first consulted spiritual or traditional healers in over two-thirds (69%) of cases compared to 17.4% who consulted psychiatrists and 13.8% who consulted a GP. A study of south-eastern Nigeria (Odinka et al., 2014) found that while 61.1% and 14.7% of the sample initially took the spiritual and traditional pathways respectively, only 9.2% took the biomedical pathway. A study of south-southern Nigeria reported that patients initially consulted more religious (48%) and traditional (20%) healers compared to a GP/Psychiatrist (12%) (Jack-Ide, Makoro, & Azibiri, 2013). While over two-thirds (69%) of patients visited religious healers, 28% consulted traditional healers, and 24% consulted GPs in a study of Northern Nigeria, none of the patients initially consulted a psychiatrist (Aghukwa, 2012).

In a study of Uganda (East Africa), Nsereko and colleagues (2011) found that traditional healers were usually the first source of care people sought when faced with mental health problems, and frequently the only source of care sought. A study of an Ethiopian sample (Bekele, Flisher, Alem, & Bahiretebeb, 2009) found that 41% of patients directly contacted a mental hospital while the rest (59%) sought care from up to four different alternative caregivers before arriving at the psychiatric hospital, with 30.9% of these consulting spiritual care providers. Another study of an Ethiopian sample found that half of the patients sought traditional treatment from either a religious healer (30.2%) or a herbalist (20.1%) before they presented at the hospital, while approximately a third (35.2%) directly sought specialised psychiatric treatment (Girma & Tesfaye, 2011).

However, in Zimbabwe, southern Africa, Patel and colleagues (1995) reported that biomedical care providers were the most commonly consulted in the first instance. Similarly, private sector GPs were mostly contacted (38.1%) in first episode cases in South Africa, followed by the police (23.8%), the public sector general medical services (14.2%), mental health practitioners (9.5%), and traditional/religious healers (9.5%) (Temmingh & Oosthuizen, 2008). Sixty per cent of respondents in a study of KwaZulu – Natal, South Africa, took the biomedical pathway as their first line of care while 40% took alternative care pathways (Mkize & Uys, 2004).

As is evident from the foregoing studies, research on pathways to mental healthcare in sub-Saharan Africa dealt mostly with clinical samples that eventually presented at biomedical psychiatric services where the customary pathway culminates. This creates a significant gap in knowledge since the pathways taken by many distressed persons do not lead to or end at such formal services. To plug this gap, Ikwuka (2016) investigated the preferred pathways to mental healthcare of non-clinical respondents, using south-eastern Nigeria as a case study. While the study found mixed treatment preferences as more than half of the respondents endorsed each of the three (traditional, spiritual, biomedical) treatment models, curiously, it found a significant preference for the biomedical (92.8%) compared to the spiritual (66.4%) and the traditional (54.4%) treatment pathways.

The findings corroborate a study of non-clinical UK-based samples which discovered that young Nigerian respondents favoured biomedical interventions and supportive environments as treatment models more than their British counterparts (Furnham & Igboaka, 2007). These findings could be interpreted as reflecting a paradigm shift from pre-scientific and spiritual conceptualisations of mental illness to an increasing scientific understanding, based possibly on improved mental health literacy. But that would be simplistic. A more complex scenario might be at play, given that behaviours are triggered by a complex interaction of attitudes, values, and situational variables (Wong, 1997). For instance, the finding may suggest a discrepancy between attitude (high endorsement of biomedical psychiatry in a non-clinical situation) and behaviour (actual patronage of a care provider in clinical situations).

As symptom severity is a major determinant of help-seeking (Biddle, Gunnel, Sharp, & Donovan, 2004), clinical samples would tend to be more pragmatic. As earlier noted (see Chapter 7, Mental Health Literacy), when the mostly uninformed families are faced with the mostly unforeseen onset of mental illness, featuring possibly bizarre psychotic symptoms, fuelled by the deeply religious worldview of the people, such a 'strange' occurrence would naturally attract a supernatural causal attribution which would also undermine the effectiveness of biomedical psychiatry. The majority of respondents in the earlier cited studies of clinical samples (Aniebue & Ekwueme, 2009; Odinka et al. 2014) who initially took the spiritual care pathway affirmed in their submission that the reason for their initial choice was a belief that the illness was due to supernatural factors and their confidence in the spiritual care pathway.

Crisis occurs when previous coping methods can no longer solve problems and, in such situations, people are more receptive and apt to change (Donnelly, 2005). As Angermeyer and colleagues (2001) observed, if initial treatment experiences fail, the formal expert system is clearly favoured. This reflects the temporality of pathways to care. Thus, help-seeking stages are not necessarily sequential or discrete, with individuals sometimes describing their getting help for a mental health problem as simply 'muddling through' (Cauce et al., 2002). In the context of the developing world, a help-seeking process can start with any one of traditional, faith or biomedical healer and end with another, with the possibility of passing through all the pathways or even involving a syncretic mix of therapies.

Dinos and colleagues (2017) reported the case of a 55-year-old Nigerian man (FN) who belonged to a Christian Pentecostal religious group. FN suffered from Schizoaffective Disorder and was brought to a hospital for an acute relapse characterised by auditory hallucinations of religious content, agitation, hyperactivity, elated mood, religious delusions, and formal thought disorder bordering on a confusional state. He also displayed disorganised and chaotic behaviours such as defecating in the ward corridor and stripping naked in public spaces. After six weeks of insufficient improvement following generous doses of psychotropic medications, his wife requested a consultation with the treating team. She stated that she was well aware of the diagnosis of Schizoaffective Disorder and the importance of regular compliance with medications which had sustained her husband for many years.

However, besides the symptoms of the mental condition, she could also detect clear signs of spirit possession, for example, when her husband claimed to be able to hear the voices of deceased family members. She asked the treating team to address the clinical symptomatology more aggressively with psychotropic medications so that when her husband was "mentally stronger" she would be able to bring in their pastor for a religious healing ceremony. She believed it was the psychotic relapse that increased her husband's vulnerability to spirit possession, hence her requests to the medical team to address the former in order for her to be able to address the latter. Rogler and Hollingshead (1985) cited a case in Puerto Rico where a man prone to outbreaks of violence was taken to a psychiatrist by relatives so that he could be tranquilised and then taken to a "genuine" therapist, a spiritualist medium. The correspondence between need and action is, therefore, neither direct nor reliable and the cessation of a pathway need not empirically coincide with the termination of the problem. Ultimately, however, pathways are travelled in the hope of attaining secure services which may be reached in formal or informal settings.

The social desirability factor could also inform discrepancies between attitude and behaviour. The perceived efficacy of biomedical psychiatry notwithstanding, a 'colonial mentality' is still evident in sub-Saharan Africa – the thinking that foreign (Western) products are superior to their local alternatives. Such a mindset is further reinforced in mental healthcare in the seeming 'imperialisation' of mental health as evident, for instance, in the Western creation of official categories of mental illnesses; the Diagnostic and Statistical Manual of Mental Disorders (DSM) and the International Classification of Diseases (ICD) which have become worldwide standards. The panels that finalise these diagnostic categories are unrepresentative of the global population. For instance, only two of the 47 psychiatrists who contributed to the initial draft of the World Health Organisation's diagnostic system (ICD-10) were from Africa, and none of the 14 field trial centres were located in sub-Saharan Africa (White, 2013).

Such biases also impose methodological limitations to pathway studies whereby contacts with alternative services are usually underreported (Lincoln & McGorry, 1995), possibly because of the perception that informal contacts do not warrant equal status on the help-seeking pathway. Identifying with the 'superior' Western model would therefore be the more socially acceptable choice to make, especially by non-clinical respondents who are not under the pressure of symptom severity and who would therefore have the luxury of responding according to which behaviours are socially desirable. In a related Indian study (Kulhara, Avasthi & Sharma, 2000), although only 33% of respondents endorsed that magico-religious treatments could improve the patient's condition, in reality, the pathway was taken in 58% of the cases.

Socially desirable responses could furthermore be fuelled in the region by the increasingly bad press and credibility questions faced by spiritual and traditional care providers. While these are characteristically exaggerated in the virtual world of the home videos, including the hugely popular Nigerian (Nollywood) and Ghanaian movie industries, genuine concerns have also been raised. For instance, writing in the Guardian UK on December 9, 2007, Tracy McVeigh notes that "the Evangelical pastors are helping to create a terrible new campaign of violence against young Nigerians. Innocent children and babies, branded as evil, are being abused, abandoned and even murdered while the preachers make money out of the fear of their parents and their communities .... For the most part, these so-called servants of God do nothing but peddle fear and recrimination. In a maddened state of terror, parents and whole villages turn on the child. They are burnt, poisoned, slashed, chained to the trees, buried alive or simply beaten and chased off into the bush." Similarly, in Thisday Newspaper of May 7, 2014, the leading columnist Eniola Bello described the 'miracle-working' pastors pervasive in the Nigerian Pentecostal genre as 'merchandising miracles'.

Meanwhile, projecting the triumphalism of Christianity, faith healers take their rivalry with the traditional healers to the home video screens where many Evangelical Churches sponsor proselytising movies that associate traditional medicine with diabolism and excessive blood rituals, thus making it socially abhorrent. Hence, the traditional pathway is made to appear obsolete and unfashionable, which explains why this pathway is mostly taken nocturnally. The case for the traditional pathway is further not helped by the belief that, though people could access it to get cures for their ailments and prophylactics against future misfortunes, some could do so to seek diabolical means to harm other people (Mulatu, 1999). It must be recognised, though, that contempt for native systems has a structural link with the historical colonial demonisation and subsequent banning of African traditional beliefs and practices.

Yet, the fact that more than half of the respondents in the case study of south-eastern Nigeria (Ikwuka, 2016) endorsed spiritual and traditional care in spite of the foregoing, only goes to further underscore how deeply socio-cultural and religious norms, beliefs, and values shape the manner in which the people in the region conceptualise and respond to experiences including psychopathology.

12 Conclusion

Towards a Complementary Model of Mental Healthcare

Studies indicate an increased recognition of the evidence base of biomedical care in the sub-Saharan African region. As Hugo and colleagues (2003) noted, while there is certainly a case that the concept of "a pill for every ill" should not be fostered, it is increasingly clear that medication plays a crucial role in containing the symptoms of serious disorders such as schizophrenia. Clients in a South African study who expressed satisfaction with the treatment they received in district hospitals and mental health institutions, based their contentment on the significant reduction of the symptoms they experienced following medication (Mkize, & Uys, 2004). However, questions have been raised regarding the extent to which biomedical psychiatric outcomes are culturally sensitive and inclusive (see also Chapter 7, Cultural (In)appropriateness of Care).

On the other hand, while traditional and faith healers may play an important role in addressing mental health needs by offering culturally responsive treatments (Abbo, 2011; Shibre, Spangeus, Henriksson, Negash, & Jacobsson, 2008), these pathways are associated with the longest delay in patients reaching specialised services, hence the longer duration of untreated illness (Gureje, Acha, & Odejide, 1995; Sorsdahl, Stein, & Flisher, 2013). While the median time taken to reach specialist mental health services in Australia following the biomedical pathway was six months, with a significantly shorter time for patients with psychotic disorders (Steel et al., 2006), the median delay between the onset of illness and arrival at the psychiatric hospital in a study of an Ethiopian sample was three years and two weeks (Bekele, Flisher, Alem, & Bahiretebeb, 2009). A study of a Nigerian sample (Adeosun, Adegbohun, Adewumi, & Jeje, 2013) found that patients who first consulted GPs presented to an average of one care provider before presenting to mental health professionals, while those who consulted alternative services saw an average of six care providers before presenting to mental health professionals. While service users initiated contact with traditional/spiritual healers within one month after the onset of symptoms in the study, biomedical psychiatric facilities were not consulted until about nine months later.

A study of Northern Nigeria found that none of the patients first consulted a psychiatrist in the care pathway and the mean length of illness before psychiatric evaluation was four and a half years (Aghukwa, 2012). Delays are increased by the lack of referral skills on the part of traditional and spiritual care providers. This may be informed by the conception of referral as an admission of incompetence. Furthermore, as earlier noted (see Chapter 8, Social Network), although a study (Bonin, Fournier, & Blais, 2007) hinted that limited social networks predicted the restricted utilisation of mental health resources, research also hinted at the irony of the inhibitory influence of tightly meshed social networks that can insulate individuals from linking up with health facilities.

The foregoing thus demonstrates that no healthcare model is self-sufficient, nor are different models equally capable of rendering help quantitatively or qualitatively. Practitioners and policymakers must, therefore, not assume homogeneity of approach to mental health care across cultures. It reinforces the call of the UN Permanent Forum on Indigenous Issues (2014) for a complementary approach to healthcare that envisages consultation with, referral to, or joint therapy with trained spiritual and traditional practitioners.

Biomedical and alternative healers could help persons with mental illness by resolving different issues relating to the same illness. For instance, following Litwak's (1968) formulation, traditional kinship structures, resting on permanent relationships, can support long-term commitments to care. Friendship ties, resting on free choice and affectivity, can support the provision of new information. Based on geographical proximity, neighbours can deal with emergencies while biomedical psychiatric institutions, resting on trained expertise and concentrated resources, can provide specialised segmented services. Indeed, the strong social network characteristic of the traditional pathway could complement the impersonal setting of biomedical psychiatric care where the patient, already alienated by the condition, is expected to bare the inner turmoil of their private life to a virtual stranger of, usually, a higher social class. Thornicroft (2008) had observed that Blacks especially are more likely to seek help if their families are supportive and if a family member has had a positive personal experience of mental healthcare.

Moreover, since patients with psychosis present early to traditional and faith healers in the developing world, constructive engagement with these alternative care providers will be indispensable in achieving early referral to specialised services. In this regard, dialogue needs to proceed with openness and objectivity that allows for the possibility of cross-referral whereby the biomedical psychiatric model could, for instance, defer to the traditional model, especially when conditions are scientifically inexplicable, as could happen with culture-related phenomena about which it has been observed that biomedical psychiatry has no satisfactory response

(Roe & Swarbrick, 2007). Indeed, studies suggest that a significant number of patients presenting at primary care services are diagnosed with medically unexplained (somatoform) symptoms (Kirmayer, Groleau, Looper, & Dominicé, 2004). Many of these symptoms have a cultural basis and incorporate or are mediated by cultural beliefs and idioms of distress (Bhui & Dinos, 2008). The prospect of cross-referral would demonstrate to the alternative care providers that the practice of referral is not an admission of incompetence but a valuable and commendable skill.

Indigenous psychiatrists recognise the need to educate and integrate spiritual and traditional healers into the mainstream biomedical mental health services for maximised service delivery (Yusuf, 2010). When offered a choice between biomedical, traditional, or combined treatment should they develop mental illness, a third of respondents in the study of Primary Health Care workers in south-western Nigeria had opted for combined treatment (Ogunlesi & Adelekan, 1988). This mirrors the findings of the case study of south-eastern Nigeria (Ikwuka, 2016) that equally reflected a preference for a mix of biomedical, spiritual, and traditional healing methods. This was reinforced by the finding also of mixed causal attributions for mental illness with biological, psychosocial, and supernatural causations endorsed almost in equal measure. This was further strengthened by the positive relationship found between the three causal models. These reflect the worldview whereby cultural conceptions of the mind remain interwoven with a variety of cultural and religious beliefs as well as the ecological and social world. They underscore the complexity of life in traditional and borderline societies that live harmoniously with experiences that could border on contradictions when considered from the perspective of Western psychology and psychiatry (see Chapter 7, The Sociocultural Context).

To achieve therapeutic alliances and meet cultural expectations of outcomes in these societies, healthcare providers must not insist on a linear or 'logical' (Western) approaches to care, which could alienate sufferers. This becomes all the more pertinent in the face of the globalisation of Western culture, which presents just one version of human nature – one set of ideas about pain and suffering – as being definitive. Adopting a strictly Western approach in these cultural contexts could strip away the local beliefs that provide buffers and safe harbour in the face of crises. It would be culturally inappropriate, for instance, to hurry to conclusive terminal diagnosis in a sociocultural context that believes that 'nothing is impossible with God'. Writing on the emergence of Post-Traumatic Stress Disorder (PTSD) as a symptom of a troubled post-modern world, Bracken (2001), observed the move away from religious and other belief systems which offered individuals stable pathways through life and meaningful frameworks with which to encounter suffering and death.

The classic case of Mr B in the UK's National Health Services comes to mind. Mr B, a 73-year-old man with mental illness, had a life-threatening leg infection. Doctors ruled that amputation was indispensable to save his life, but Mr B declined the operation. This could have sufficed legally, save for the fact that Mr B lacked 'mental capacity'. The operation would have left him dependent in a nursing home, an idea which he detested, and he also loathed the prospect of living with the bitter memory of having been compelled to undergo major surgery against his wish. Mr B declared that he was not afraid to die, that he knew where he was going and that the angels had told him that he was going to heaven which he considered a better life than the one he was presently living.

The NHS Trust argued that Mr B's wishes, feelings and religious beliefs should be disregarded because they were closely connected with his mental illness. After meeting with Mr B, the judge disagreed with the NHS Trust and granted his plea to refuse amputation. The judge noted that his religious beliefs were deeply meaningful to him and did not deserve to be trivialised as delusions; they were his faith, and they were an intrinsic part of who he was. The judge was impressed by Mr B's force of personality. After a difficult life, marked by loneliness, disappointments and repeated setbacks, Mr B had fierce independence that could not be ignored. The judge concluded that it would not be in Mr B's interest to take away his little remaining independence and dignity for the sake of a traumatic and uncertain struggle that he and no one else would have had to endure. The judge observed moreover that his fortitude in the face of death; however, he had come by it, would be the envy of many people in better mental health (Hitchens, 2015).

The foregoing underscores the imperative of evolving an integrated model of healthcare that is sensitive to the spiritual and cultural needs of the people. Ignoring the beliefs of clients could cause psychiatry to miss an important psychological and social factor that may either be a powerful resource for healing or a major cause of pathology (Koenig, 2008). Complementary approaches to care have worked effectively in a southern African (Lesotho) context (Obioha, & Molale, 2011) and equally in Europe (Sevilla-Dedieu et al., 2010). In an imaginative programme in Hungary, pastors train alongside mental health professionals because of the observed link between people's mental health, religion, and spirituality (Tomcsanyi, 2000). Pakistan equally exemplifies an innovative and comprehensive strategy, specifically designed to take advantage of local opportunities, to meet some of the challenges faced in developing countries. The strategy includes collaborating with traditional healers who have received some training, leading to increased identification and professional referral of individuals with mental disorders (Rahman, Mubbashar, Gater, & Goldberg, 1998).

The need for cooperation with indigenous models received a further boost with the findings of three cross-national studies by the World Health Organisation: the International Pilot Study of Schizophrenia (IPSS) (World Health Organization, 1979), the Determinants of Outcome of Severe Mental Disorder (DOSMeD) (Jablensky et al., 1992), and their sequel, the International Study of Schizophrenia (ISoS) (Harrison et al., 2001). These suggest arguably that schizophrenia has a better prognosis in indigenous (non-industrialised) societies.

While the pragmatics of complementary care must be determined, training to promote the improved cultural competency of local mental health professionals would be a good starting point towards a bottom-up approach that recognises the importance of local conceptualisations of mental health difficulties for optimal service delivery. Cultural competency entails an understanding of people's rules for behaviour, language, religion, history, traditional beliefs, and values (Cross, Bazron, Dennis, & Isaacs, 1989). It enables professionals to be more empathetic and forge therapeutic alliances with clients.

Campinha-Bacote (2002) identified five components of cultural competence to include: *awareness*, or sensitivity to the values and lifestyles of clients; *knowledge*, or mastery of information about alternative world-views, as well as biogenetic variations among groups; *skill*, or a collection of relevant data regarding health problems; *encounter*, or face-to-face meetings with diverse peoples; and *desire*, or the motivation to ally with patients. Comprehensive reviews of literature reveal that increased cultural competence significantly improves patient satisfaction with treatment, and participants undergoing cultural competence programmes showed significant gains in knowledge about and attitudes toward culturally different groups (Beach et al., 2005; Price et al., 2005).

To facilitate therapy, causal theories and prescriptions for cure need to be meaningful to the patient in terms of the realities they understand. If patients do not believe in the theories of the cause and/or cure advanced for their condition, it may affect treatment adherence and follow-up. The significance of an inductive bottom-up approach to care is such that how a people in a culture conceptualise mental illness – how they categorise and prioritise the symptoms, attempt to heal them, and set expectations for their course and outcome influences the diseases themselves (Watters, 2010). A culturally competent professional would allay the fears of potential clients that they may be misdiagnosed or their beliefs and values dismissively pathologised. Moreover, a culturally competent professional would be better placed to recognise and intervene when beliefs are indeed becoming pathological. Such a professional would be decisive for the complementary model that envisages consultation with, a referral to, or joint therapy with trained spiritual and traditional service providers.

References

Abasiubong, F., Obembe, A., & Ekpo, E. (2008). The opinion and attitude of mothers to mental retardation in Lagos, Nigeria. *Nigerian Journal of Psychiatry*, 6(2), 80–85.

Abasiubong, F., Ekott, J. U., & Bassey, E. A. (2007). A comparative study of attitude to mental illness between journalists and nurses in Uyo, Nigeria. *African Journal of Medicine and Medical Sciences*, 36, 345–351.

Abayomi, O., Adelufosi, A. O., & Olajide, A. (2013). Changing attitude to mental illness among community mental health volunteers in south-western Nigeria. *International Journal of Social Psychiatry*, 59, 609–612.

Abbo, C. (2011). Profiles and outcome of traditional healing practices for severe mental illnesses in two districts of Eastern Uganda. *Global Health Action*, 4, 1.

Abbo, C., Okello, E., Ekblad, S., Waako, P., & Musisi, S. (2008). Lay concepts of psychosis in Busoga, Eastern Uganda: A pilot study. *World Cultural Psychiatry Research Review*, 3(3), 132–145.

Abdullah, T., & Brown, T. L. (2011). Mental illness stigma and ethnocultural beliefs, values, and norms: An integrative review. *Clinical Psychology Review*, 31, 934–948.

Abdulmalik, J. O., & Sale, S. (2012). Pathways to psychiatric care for children and adolescents at a tertiary facility in northern Nigeria. *Journal of Public Health in Africa*, 3, 15–17.

Abiodun, O. A. (1991). Knowledge and attitude concerning mental health of primary health care workers in Nigeria. *The International Journal of Social Psychiatry*, 37, 113–120.

Addis, M. E., & Mahalik, J. R. (2003). Men, masculinity, and the contexts of help seeking. *American Psychologist*, 58, 5–14.

Adebiyi, A. O., Fagbola, M. A., Olakehinde, O., & Ogunniyi, A. (2015). Enacted and implied stigma for dementia in a community in south-west Nigeria. *Psychogeriatrics*, 16, 268–273.

Adeola, O. O., Babatunde, A., & Olayinka, O. O. (2017). Effect of a mental health training programme on Nigerian school pupils' perceptions of mental illness. *Child and Adolescent Psychiatry and Mental Health*, 11, 19.

Adeosun, I. I., Adegbohun, A. A., Adewumi, T. A., & Jeje, O. O. (2013). The pathways to the first contact with mental health services among patients with schizophrenia in Lagos, Nigeria. *Schizophrenia Research and Treatment*, 769161, 1–8.

Adesomoju, A. (2013, June 14). Lagos: 21-Year-old arraigned for sleeping with mentally ill inmates. *Punch Newspapers.* Retrieved from http://www.punchng. com/metro/21-year-old-arraigned-for-sleeping-with-mentally-ill-inmates/.

Adewuya, A. O., & Makanjuola, R. O. (2008). Lay beliefs regarding causes of mental illness in Nigeria: Pattern and correlates. *Social Psychiatry and Psychiatric Epidemiology*, 43(4), 336–341.

Adewuya A. O., & Makanjuola, R. O. (2009). Preferred treatment for mental illness among south-western Nigerians. *Psychiatric Services*, 60(1), 121–124.

Adewuya, A. O., & Oguntade, A. A. (2007). Doctors' attitude towards people with mental illness in western Nigeria. *Social Psychiatry & Psychiatric Epidemiology*, 42, 931–936.

Adewuya, A. O., Owoeye, A. O., Erinfolami, A. O., & Ola, B. A. (2011). Correlates of self-stigma among outpatients with mental illness in Lagos, Nigeria. *International Journal of Social Psychiatry*, 57(4), 418–427.

Addison, S. J., & Thorpe, S. J. (2004). Factors involved in the formation of attitudes towards those who are mentally ill. *Social Psychiatry and Psychiatric Epidemiology*, 39, 228–234.

Adler, A. K., & Wahl, O. F. (1998). Children's beliefs about people labelled mentally ill. *American Journal of Orthopsychiatry*, 68, 321–326.

Adler, L. L., & Mukherji, B. R. (1995). *Spirit versus scalpel: Traditional healing and modem psychotherapy.* Westport, CT: Bergin & Garvey.

Afana, A., Dalgard, O., Bjertness, E., Grunfled, B., & El-Sarraj, E. (2000). The attitude of Palestinian primary healthcare professionals in the Gaza strip towards mental illness. *Egyptian Journal of Psychiatry*, 23, 101–111.

Afolayan, J. A., & Okpemuza, M. (2011). Sociocultural factors affecting mental health service delivery in neuropsychiatric hospital, Port Harcourt, Rivers State, Nigeria. *Continental Journal of Nursing Science* 3(1), 31–40.

Agara, A. J., & Makanjuola, A. B. (2006). Pattern and pathways of psychiatric presentation at the out-patient clinic of a Neuro-Psychiatric Hospital in Nigeria. *Nigerian Journal of Psychiatry*, 4(1), 30–37.

Agbodike, C. (2008). *A centenary of catholic missionary activities in Ihiala 1908–2008.* Nkpor, Nigeria: Globe Communications.

Aghukwa, N. C. (2009a). Attitude of health workers to the care of psychiatric patients. *Annals of General Psychiatry*, 8(1), 19.

Aghukwa, N. C. (2009b). Secondary school teachers' attitude to mental illness in Ogun state, Nigeria. *African Journal of Psychiatry*, 12(1), 59–63.

Aghukwa N. C. (2010). Attitudes towards psychiatry of undergraduate medical students at Bayero University, Nigeria. *South African Journal of Psychiatry*, 16, 147–152.

Aghukwa, C. N. (2012). Care seeking and beliefs about the cause of mental illness among Nigerian psychiatric patients and their families. *Psychiatric Services*, 63(6), 616–618.

Ahmed, S., Adams, A., Chowdhury, M., & Bhuiya, A. (2000). Gender, socioeconomic development and health-seeking behaviour in Bangladesh. *Social Science and Medicine*, 51(3), 361–371.

Aina, O. F. (2004). Mental illness and cultural issues in West African films: Implications for orthodox psychiatric practice. *Medical Humanities*, 30, 23–26.

Aina, O. F., Oshodi, O. Y., Erinfolami, A. R., Adeyemi, J. D., & Suleiman, T. F. (2015). Non-mental health workers' attitudes and social distance towards people with mental illness in a Nigerian teaching hospital. *South Sudan Medical Journal*, 8(3), 57–59.

Akinkuotu, E., & Aworinde, T. (2019, May 19). Rising suicide crisis: How 250 psychiatrists battle Nigeria's 60 million mental cases. *Punch Newspapers*. Retrieved from https://punchng.com/rising-suicide-crisis-how-250-psychiatrists-battle-nigerias-60-million-mental-cases/.

Al-Darmaki, F. R. (2003). Attitudes towards seeking professional psychological help: What really counts for United Arab Emirates University students? *Social Behavior and Personality*, 31(5), 497–508.

Alegria, M., Robles, R., Freeman, D. H., Vera, M., Jiménez, A. L., Ríos, C., & Ríos, R. (1991). Patterns of mental health utilization among island Puerto Rican poor. *American Journal of Public Health*, 81(7), 875–879.

Alexander, L. A., & Link, B. G. (2003). The impact of contact on stigmatizing attitudes toward people with mental illness. *Journal of Mental Health*, 12(3), 271–289.

Al-Krenawi, A., & Graham, J. R. (2000). Culturally sensitive social work practice with Arab clients in mental health settings. *Health and Social Work*, 25(1), 9–22.

Al-Krenawi, A., Graham, J. R., Al-Bedah, E. A., Kadri, H. M., & Sehwail, M. A. (2009). Cross-national comparison of Middle Eastern university students: Help-seeking behaviors, attitudes toward helping professionals, and cultural beliefs about mental health problems. *Community Mental Health Journal*, 45, 26–36.

Al-Krenawi, A., & Graham, J. R. (2011). Mental health help-seeking among Arab university students in Israel, differentiated by religion. *Mental Health, Religion & Culture*, 14(2), 157–167.

Al-Rowaie, O. O. (2005). *Predictors of attitudes toward seeking professional psychological help among Kuwait University Students* (Doctoral thesis, Virginia Polytechnic Institute and State University, Blacksburg, Virginia). Retrieved from https://vtechworks.lib.vt.edu/bitstream/handle/10919/30166/OdahPhD_Ch1.pdf.

Alzubaidi, A., Baluch, B., & Moafi, A. (1996). Attitudes toward the mentally disabled in a non-Western society. *Journal of Social Behaviour & Personality*, 10, 933–938.

American Psychiatric Association. (2018, June 24). People: African Americans. Retrieved June from http://www.psychiatry.org/african-americans.

American Psychiatric Association. (2013). *Diagnostic and statistical manual of mental disorder* (5th ed.). Washington, DC: Publisher.

American Psychological Association. (2018, August 2). Teaching tip sheet: Stigma and prejudice. Retrieved from http://www.apa.org/pi/aids/resources/education/stigma-prejudice.aspx.

Anderson, K. K., Fuhrer, R., & Malla, A. K. (2010). The pathways to mental health care of first-episode psychosis patients: A systematic review. *Psychological Medicine*, 40, 1585–1597.

Andrade, L., Caraveo-Anduaga, J. J., Berglund, P., Bijl, R., Kessler, R. C., Demler, O., … Wittchen, H.-U. (2000). Cross-national comparisons of the prevalences and correlates of mental disorders. *Bulletin of the World Health Organization*, 78, 413–425.

Angel, R., & Thoits, P. (1987). The impact of culture on the cognitive structure of illness. *Culture, Medicine & Psychiatry*, 11, 465–494.

Angermeyer, M. C., Buyantugs, L., Kenzine, D. V., & Matschinger, H. (2004). Effects of labeling on public attitudes towards people with schizophrenia: Are there cultural differences? *Acta Psychiatrica Scandinavica*, 109, 420–425.

Angermeyer, M. C., & Dietrich, S. (2006). Public beliefs about and attitudes towards people with mental illness: A review of population studies. *Acta Psychiatrica Scandinavica*, 113, 163–179.

Angermeyer, M. C., Holzinger, A., & Matschinger, H. (2009). Mental health literacy and attitude towards people with mental illness: A trend analysis based on population surveys in the eastern part of Germany. *European Psychiatry*, 24, 225–232.

Angermeyer, M. C., & Matschinger, H. (1996). Public attitude towards psychiatric treatment. *Acta Psychiatrica Scandinavica*, 94, 326–336.

Angermeyer, M. C., & Matschinger, H. (1997). Social distance towards the mentally ill: Results of representative surveys in the Federal Republic of Germany. *Psychological Medicine*, 27, 131–141.

Angermeyer, M. C., & Matschinger, H. (2004). Public attitudes towards psychotropic drugs: Have there been any changes in recent years? *Pharmacopsychiatry*, 37, 152–156.

Angermeyer, M. C., Matschinger, H., & Corrigan, P. W. (2004). Familiarity with mental illness and social distance from people with schizophrenia and major depression: Testing a model using data from a representative population survey. *Schizophrenia Research*, 69(2–3), 175–182.

Angermeyer, M. C., Matschinger, H., & Riedel-Heller, S. G. (2001). What to do about mental health disorder – help seeking recommendations of the lay public. *Acta Psychiatrica Scandinavica*, 103, 220–225.

Angermeyer, M. C., & Schulze, B. (2001). Reinforcing stereotypes: How the focus on forensic cases in news reporting may influence public attitudes towards the mentally ill. *International Journal of Law and Psychiatry*, 24, 469–486.

Aniebue, P., & Ekwueme, C. (2009). Health-seeking behaviour of mentally ill patients in Enugu, Nigeria. *South African Journal of Psychiatry*, 15(1), 19–22.

Antonak, R. F., & Harth, R. (1994). Psychometric analysis and revision of the Mental Retardation Attitude Inventory. *Mental Retardation*, 32, 272–280.

Anyebe, E. E., Olisah, V. O., Garba, S. N., Amedu, M. (2019). Current status of mental health services at the primary healthcare level in Northern Nigeria. *Administration and Policy in Mental Health and Mental Health Services Research*, 46(5), 620–628.

Appleby, L., Mortensen P. B., & Faragher, B. E. (1998). Suicide and other causes of morality after post-partum psychiatric admission. *The British Journal of Psychiatry*, 173(9), 209–211.

Appleby, L., & Wessely, S. (1988). Public attitudes to mental illness: The influence of the Hungerford massacre. *Medicine, Science and the Law*, 28, 291–295.

Arboleda-Florez, J. (1998). Mental illness and violence: An epidemiological appraisal of the evidence. *Canadian Journal of Psychiatry*, 43, 989–996.

Arboleda-Flórez, J. (2001). Stigmatization and human rights violations. In *World Health Organization, Mental Health: A Call for Action by World Health Ministers* (pp. 57–70). Geneva: World Health Organization.

Aroyewun-Adekomaiya, K., & Aroyewun, T. F. (2019). Representation of mental illness in movies: A Nigerian perspective. *African Journal for the Psychological Study of Social Issues*, 22(2), 103–117.

Arvaniti, A., Samakouri, M., Kalamara, E., Bochtsou, V., Bikos., C., & Livaditis, M. (2009). Health service staff's attitudes towards patients with mental illness. *Social Psychiatry & Psychiatric Epidemiology*, 44, 658–665.

Asenso-Okyere, W., Anum, A., Osei-Akoto., I., & Adukonu, A. (1998). Cost recovery in Ghana: Are there any changes in health seeking behaviour? *Health Policy and Planning*, 13, 181–188.

Asuni, T., Schoenberg, F., & Swift, C. (Eds.). (1994). *Mental health and disease in Africa*. Ibadan, Nigeria: Spectrum Books Ltd.

Atilola, O. (2015). Level of community mental health literacy in sub-Saharan Africa: Current studies are limited in number, scope, spread, and cognizance of cultural nuances. *Nordic Journal of Psychiatry*, 69, 93–101.

Atilola, O., & Olayiwola, F. (2011). Mind frames in Nollywood: Frames of mental illness in Nigerian home videos. *Research Journal of Medical Sciences*, 5(3), 166–171.

Aubrey, R. (1991). International students on campus: A challenge for counselors, medical providers, and clinicians. *Smith College Students in Social Work*, 62, 20–33.

Austin, A., & Goodman, R. (2017). The impact of social connectedness and internalized transphobic stigma on self-esteem among transgender and gender non-conforming adults. *Journal of Homosexuality*, 64(6), 825–841.

Australia Department of Health and Aged Care. (1998). *Mental health promotion and prevention: National action plan under the second national mental health plan: 1998–2003*. Canberra: Promotion and Prevention Section, Mental Health Branch, Commonwealth Department of Health and Aged Care.

Australian Nurses Federation. (2003). Survey reveals extent of violence toward nurses. *Australian Nursing Journal*, 11, 9.

Awojobi, A. O. (2011). Rejuvenating primary health care in Nigeria – The Ibarapa Experience. *Paper presented at the symposium organized by the editorial board of DOKITA Paul Hendrickse Lecture Theatre*. University College Hospital, Ibadan, Nigeria.

Ay, P., Save, D., & Fidanoglu, O. (2006). Does stigma concerning mental disorders differ through medical education? A survey among medical students in Istanbul. *Social Psychiatry and Psychiatric Epidemiology*, 41, 63–67.

Aydin, N., Yigit, A., Inandi, T., & Kirpinar, I. (2003). Attitudes of hospital staff toward mentally ill patients in a teaching hospital, Turkey. *International Journal of Social Psychiatry*, 49(1), 17–26.

Ayorinde, O., Gureje, O., & Lawal, R. (2004). Psychiatric research in Nigeria: Bridging tradition and modernisation. *British Journal of Psychiatry*, 184, 536–538.

Bag, B., Yilmaz, S., & Kirpinar, I. (2006). Factors influencing social distance from people with schizophrenia. *International Journal of Clinical Practice*, 60, 289–294.

Baibabayev, A., Cunningham, D., de Jong, K. (2000). Update on the state of mental health in Tajikistan. *Mental Health Reforms*, 5, 14–16.

Bailey, S. (1998). An exploration of critical care nurses' and doctors' attitudes toward psychiatric patients. *Australian Journal of Advanced Nursing*, 15(3), 8–14.

Barimah, K. B., & Teijlingen, E. R. V. (2008). The use of traditional medicine by Ghanaians in Canada. *BMC Complementary and Alternative Medicine*, 8(1), 30.

Barker, G., Olukoya, A., & Aggleton, P. (2005). Young people, social support and help-seeking. *International Journal of Adolescent Medicine and Health*, 17(4), 315–335.

Barksdale, C. L., & Molock, S. D. (2008). Perceived norms and mental health help seeking among African American college students. *Journal of Behavioral Health Services and Research*, 36(3), 285–299.

Barney, L. J., Griffiths, K. M., Jorm, A. F., & Christensen, H. (2006). Stigma about depression and its impact on help-seeking intentions. *Australian and New Zealand Journal of Psychiatry*, 40(1), 51–54.

Baruth, L. G., & Manning, M. L. (2003). *Multicultural counseling and psychotherapy: A lifespan perspective.* Upper Saddle River, NJ: Merrill Prentice Hall.

Battaglia, J., Coverdale, J. H., & Bushong, C. P. (1990). Evaluation of a mental illness awareness week program in public schools. *American Journal of Psychiatry*, 147, 324–329.

Beach, M. C., Price, E. G., Gary, T. L., Robinson, K. A., Gozu, A., Alacio, A., ... Cooper, L. A. (2005). Cultural competence: A systematic review of health care provider educational interventions. *Medical Care*, 43, 356–373.

Bekele, Y. Y., Flisher, A. J., Alem, A., Bahiretebeb, Y. (2009). Pathways to psychiatric care in Ethiopia. *Psychological Medicine*, 39, 475–483.

Bell, J. S., Aaltonen, S. E., Bronstein, E., Desplenter, F. A., Foulon, V., Vitola, A., ... Chen, T. F. (2008). Attitudes of pharmacy students toward people with mental disorders, a six country study. *Pharmacy World and Science*, 30(5), 595–599.

Benenson, J. F., & Koulnazarian, M. (2008). Sex differences in help-seeking appear in early childhood. *British Journal of Developmental Psychology*, 26(2), 163–170.

Bergner, E., Leiner, A. S., Carter, T., Franz, L., Thompson, N. J., & Compton, M. T. (2008). The period of untreated psychosis before treatment initiation: A qualitative study of family members' perspectives. *Comprehensive Psychiatry*, 49, 530–536.

Betancourt, J. R., Green, A. R., & Carrillo, J. E. (2000). The challenge of cross-cultural healthcare-diversity, ethics, and the medical encounter. *Bioethics Forum*, 16(3), 27–32.

Betancourt, J. R., & Maina, A. (2007). *Barriers to eliminating disparities in Clinical Practice: Lessons from the IOM report "unequal treatment".* Totowa, NJ: Humana Press.

Bhana, A., Petersen, I., Baillie, K. L., & Flisher, A. J. (2010). The Mhapp Research Programme Consortium Implementing the World Health Report 2001 recommendations for integrating mental health into primary care: A situational analysis of three African countries Ghana, South Africa and Uganda. *International Review of Psychiatry*, 22(6), 599–610.

Bhugra, D. (2006). Severe mental disorder across cultures. *Acta Psychiatrica Scandinavica. Supplementum*, 113(429), 17–23.

Bhui, K., Bhugra, D., Goldberg, D., Dunn, G., & Desai, M. (2001). Cultural influences on the prevalence of common mental disorder, general practitioner's assessments and help-seeking among Punjabi and English people visiting their general practitioner. *Psychological Medicine*, 31, 815–825.

Bhui, K., & Dinos, S. (2008). Health beliefs and culture. *Disease Management & Health Outcomes*, 16(6), 411–419.

Biddle, L., Gunnel, D., Sharp, D., & Donovan J. L. (2004). Factors influencing help seeking in mentally distressed young adults: A cross-sectional survey. *British Journal of General Practice*, 54(501), 248–253.

Binitie, A. (1970). Attitude of educated Nigerians to mental illness. *Acta Psychiatrica Scandinavica*, 46, 27–46.

Björkman, T., Angelman, T., & Jönsson, M. (2008). Attitudes towards people with mental illness: A cross-sectional study among nursing staff in psychiatric and somatic care. *Scandinavian Journal of Caring Sciences*, 22(2), 170–177.

Black, K., Peters, L., Rui, Q., Whitehorn, D., & Kopala, L. C. (2001). Duration of untreated psychosis predicts treatment outcome in an early psychosis program. *Schizophrenia Research*, 47(2–3), 215–222.

Boerner, H. (2009, February 20). Mental block. *Journal of Patient Advocacy*. Retrieved from http://nnumagazine.uberflip.com/i/198030-registered-nurse-october-2009/9.

Bolman, W. M. (1968). Cross-cultural psychotherapy. *The American Journal of Psychiatry*, 124(9), 1237.

Bonin, J. P., Fournier, L., & Blais, R. (2007). Predictors of mental health service utilization by people using resources for homeless people in Canada. *Psychiatric Services*, 58, 936–941.

Bonner, G., Lowe, T., Rawcliffe, D., & Wellman, N. (2002). Trauma for all: A pilot study of the subjective experience of physical restraint for mental health in-patients and staff in the UK. *Journal of Psychiatric and Mental Health Nursing*, 9, 465–473.

Botha, U. A., Koen, L., & Niechaus, D. J. H. (2006). Perceptions of a South African schizophrenia population with regards to community attitudes towards their illness. *Social Psychology and Psychiatric Epidemiology*, 41, 619–623.

Bracken, P. J. (2001). Post-modernity and post-traumatic stress disorder. *Social Science and Medicine*, 53(6), 733–743.

Bradley, R. H., & Michael, H. (1987). Religious affiliation, attendance, and support for "pro-family" issues in the United States. *Social Forces*, 65(3), 858–882.

Braff, D. L. (1992). Reply to cognitive therapy and schizophrenia. *Schizophrenia Bulletin*, 18(1), 37–38.

Breier, P. (2000). The progress of reforms in Slovakia. *Mental Health Reforms*, 2, 2–5.

British Psychological Society. (1998). *Briefing paper No. 16: Services to Black and ethnic minority people*. Leicester: Division of Clinical Psychology, British Psychological Society.

Brockington, I. F., Hall, P., Levings, J., & Murray, C. (1993). The community's tolerance of the mentally ill. *British Journal of Psychiatry*, 162, 93–99.

Brown, L., Trujillo, L., & Macintyre, K. (2001). Interventions to reduce HIV/AJDS stigma: What have we learned? *Horizons Population Council*, 15(1), 4–6.

Brunton, K. (1997). Stigma. *Journal of Advanced Nursing*, 26, 891–898.

Budman, C. L., Lipson, J. B., & Meleis, A. I. (1992). The cultural consultant in mental health care: The case of an Arab adolescent. *American Journal of Orthopsychiatry*, 62, 359–370.

Burgess, P. M., Pirkis, J. E., Slade, T. N., Johnson, A. K., Meadows, G. N., & Gunn, J. M. (2009). Service use for mental health problems: Findings from the 2007 National Survey of Mental Health and Wellbeing. *Australian and New Zealand Journal of Psychiatry*, 43, 615–623.

Burns, J. K., & Tomita, A. (2015). Traditional and religious healers in the pathway to care for people with mental disorders in Africa: A systematic review and meta-analysis. *Social Psychiatry and Psychiatric Epidemiology*, 50, 867–877.

Burton, V. S. (1990). The consequences of official labels: A research note on rights lost by the mentally ill, mentally incompetent, and convicted felons. *Community Mental Health Journal*, 26, 267–276.

Byrne, P. (1997). Psychiatric stigma: Past, passing and to come. *Journal of the Royal Society of Medicine*, 90, 618–620.

Byrne, P. (1998). Fall and rise of the movie "psycho-killer". *Psychiatric Bulletin*, 22, 174–176.

Byrne P. (2000). Stigma of mental illness and ways of diminishing it. *Advances in Psychiatric Treatment*, 6, 65–72.

Calhoun, E. A., Whitley, E. M., Esparza, A., Ness, E., Greene, A., Garcia, R., Valverde, P. A. (2010). A national patient navigator training program. *Health Promotion Practice*, 11, 205–215.

Cameron, L., Leventhal, E. A., & Leventhal, H. (1993). Symptom representations and affect as determinants of care seeking in a community-dwelling, adult sample population. *Health Psychology*, 12, 171–179.

Campbell-Hall, V., Petersen, I., Bhana, A., Mjadu, S., Hosegood, V., & Flisher, A. J. (2010). Collaboration between traditional practitioners and primary health care staff in South Africa: Developing a workable partnership for community mental health services. *Transcultural Psychiatry*, 47(4), 610–628.

Campinha-Bacote, J. (2002). The process of cultural competence in the delivery of health care services: A model of care. *Journal of Transcultural Nursing*, 13, 181–184.

Canadian Alliance on Mental Illness and Mental Health. (2000). A call for action: Building consensus for a national plan on mental illness and mental health: Canadian alliance on mental illness and mental health. https://www.schizophrenia.ca/docs/CalltoActionCAMIMH2003English.

Canadian Mental Health Association. (1994). *Final report. Mental health anti-stigma campaign public education strategy*. Toronto: Canadian Mental Health Association, Ontario Division.

Carothers, J. C. (1948). A study of mental derangement in Africans, and an attempt to explain its peculiarities, more especially in relation to the African attitude to life. *Journal of Medical Science*, 93, 548–596.

Carrillo, J. E., Green, A. R., & Betancourt, J. R. (1999). Cross-cultural primary care: A patient-based approach. *Annals of Internal Medicine*, 130(10), 829–834.

Cauce, A. M., Domenech-Rodriguez, M., Paradise, M., Cochran, B. N., Shea, J. M., Srebnik, D., Baydar, N. (2002). Cultural and contextual influences in mental health help seeking: A focus on ethnic minority youth. *Journal of Consulting and Clinical Psychology*, 70(1), 44–55.

Chadda, R. K., Agarwal, V., Singh, M. C., & Raheja, D. (2001). Help seeking behaviour of psychiatric patients before seeking care at a mental hospital. *International Journal of Social Psychiatry*, 47(4), 471–478.

Chandra, A., & Minkovitz, C. S. (2006). Stigma starts early: Gender differences in teen willingness to use mental health services. *Journal of Adolescent Health*, 38(6), 754.e1–8.

Chandra, A., & Minkovitz, C. S. (2007). Factors that influence mental health stigma among 8th grade adolescents. *Journal of Youth and Adolescence*, 36, 763–774.

Chapman, D. P., Perry, G. S., & Strine, T. W. (2005, February 19). The vital link between chronic disease and depressive disorders: Preventing chronic disease. *Public Health Research, Practice and Policy*, 2(1). Retrieved from http://www. cdc.gov/pcd/issues/2005/jan/04_0066.htm.

Cheetham, R. W. S., & Rzadkowolski, A. (1980). Cross-cultural psychiatry and the concept of mental illness. *South African Medical Journal*, 58(8), 320–325.

Chen, S. X., Benet-Martinez, V., & Bond, M. H. (2008). Bicultural identity, bilingualism, and psychological adjustment in multicultural societies: Immigration-based and globalization-based acculturation. *Journal of Personality*, 76, 803–837.

Chew-Graham, C., Bashir, C., Chantler, K., Burman, E., & Batsleer, J. (2002). South Asian women, psychological distress and self-harm: Lessons for primary care trusts. *Health and Social Care in the Community*, 10, 339–347.

Chew-Graham, C. A., Rogers, A., & Yassin, N. (2003). 'I wouldn't want it on my CV or their records': Medical students' experiences of help-seeking for mental health problems. *Medical Education*, 37, 873–880.

Chilcot, J., Wellsted, D., & Farrington, K. (2011). Illness perceptions predict survival in haemodialysis patients. *American Journal of Nephrology*, 33, 358–363.

Chou, K. L., & Mak, K. Y. (1998). Attitudes to mental patients among Hong Kong Chinese: A trend study over two years. *International Journal of Social Psychiatry*, 44, 215–224.

Ciarrochi, J., & Deane, F. P. (2001). Emotional competence and willingness to seek help from professional and nonprofessional sources. *British Journal of Guidance and Counselling*, 29, 233–246.

Clark, L., & Hofsess, L. (1998). *Acculturation: Handbook of immigrant health*. New York: Plenum Press.

Clarke, I. (2001). *Psychosis and spirituality*. London: Whurr.

Coker, E. M. (2005). Selfhood and social distance: Toward a cultural understanding of psychiatric stigma in Egypt. *Social Science and Medicine*, 61, 920–930.

Comer, R. J. (2015). *Abnormal psychology*. London: Palgrave Macmillan.

Compton, M. T., Kaslow, N. J., & Walker, E. F. (2004). Observations on parent/ family factors that may influence the duration of untreated psychosis among African American first-episode schizophrenia-spectrum patients. *Schizophrenia Research*, 68(2–3), 373–385.

Cooper, C. L., & Swanson, N. (2002). *Workplace violence in the health sector: State of the art*. Geneva, Switzerland: International Labor Organization.

Cooper, J., & Sartorius, N. (1977). Cultural and temporal variations in schizophrenia: A speculation on the importance of industrialization. *British Journal of Psychiatry*, 130, 50–55.

Corrigan, P. W. (2004). How stigma interferes with mental health care. *American Psychologist*, 59, 614–625.

Corrigan, P. W., Druss, B. G., & Perlick, D. A. (2014). The impact of mental illness stigma on seeking and participating in mental health care. *Psychological Science in the Public Interest*, 15(2), 37–70.

Corrigan, P. W., Green, A., Lundin, R., Kubiak, M. A., & Penn, D. L. (2001). Familiarity with and social distance from people who have serious mental illness. *Psychiatric Services*, 52, 953–958.

Corrigan, P. W., Lurie, B. D., Goldman, H. H., Slopen, N., Medasani, K., & Phelan, S. (2005). How adolescents perceive the stigma of mental illness and alcohol abuse. *Psychiatric Services*, 56(5), 544–550.

Corrigan, P. W., & Miller, F. E. (2004). Shame, blame, and contamination: A review of the impact of mental illness stigma on family members. *Journal of Mental Health*, 13, 537–548.

Corrigan, P. W., & O'Shaughnessy, J. R. (2007). Changing mental illness stigma as it exists in the real world. *Australian Psychologist*, 42, 90–97.

Corrigan, P. W., & Penn, D. (1999). Lessons from social psychology on discrediting psychiatric stigma. *American Psychologist*, 54(9), 765–776.

Corrigan, P. W., & Rao, D. (2012). On the self-stigma of mental illness: Stages, disclosure, and strategies for change. *The Canadian Journal of Psychiatry*, 57(8), 464–469.

Corrigan, P. W., Rowan, D., Green, A., Lundin, R., River, P., Uphoff-Wasowski, K., ..., Kubiak, M. A. (2002). Challenging two mental illness stigmas: Personal responsibility and dangerousness. *Schizophrenia Bulletin*, 28, 293–309.

Corrigan, P. W., & Shapiro, J. (2010). Measuring the impact of programs that challenge the public stigma of mental illness. *Clinical Psychology Review*, 30, 907–922.

Corrigan, P. W., & Watson, A. C. (2002). Understanding the impact of stigma on people with mental illness. *World Psychiatry: Official Journal of the World Psychiatric Association (WPA)*, 1, 16–20.

Corrigan, P. W., Watson, A. C., Warpinski, A. C., & Gracia, G. (2004a). Implications of educating the public on mental illness, violence, and stigma. *Psychiatric Services*, 55, 577–580.

Corrigan, P. W., Watson, A. C., Warpinski, A. C., & Gracia, G. (2004b). Stigmatizing attitudes about mental illness and allocation of resources to mental health services. *Community Mental Health Journal*, 40(4), 297–307.

Corrigan, P. W., Morris, S. B., Michaels, P. J., Rafacz, J. D., & Rüsch, N. (2012). Challenging the public stigma of mental illness: A meta-analysis of outcome studies. *Psychiatric Services*, 63, 963–973.

Cotton, S., Wright, A., Harris, M. G., Jorm, A. F., & McGorry, P. D. (2006). Influence of gender on mental health literacy in young Australians. *Australian and New Zealand Journal of Psychiatry*, 40, 790–796.

Couture, S. M., & Penn, D. L. (2003). Interpersonal contact and the stigma of mental illness: A review of the literature. *Journal of Mental Health*, 12, 291–305.

Courtenay, W. H. (2000). Engendering health: A social constructionist examination of men's health beliefs and behaviours. *Psychology of Men and Masculinity*, 1, 4–15.

Cowan, S. (2003). NIMBY syndrome and public consultation policy: The implications of a discourse analysis of local responses to the establishment of a community mental health facility. *Health and Social Care in the Community*, 11(5), 379–386.

Crabb, J., Stewart, R. C., Kokota, D., Masson, N., Chabunya, S., & Krishnadas, R. (2012). Attitudes towards mental illness in Malawi: A cross-sectional survey. *BMC Public Health*, 12, 541.

Craig, M. (2004). Perinatal risk factors for neonaticide and infant homicide: Can we identify those at risk? *Journal of the Royal Society of Medicine*, 97(2), 57–61.

Crawford, P., & Brown, B. (2002). 'Like a friend going round': Reducing the stigma attached to mental healthcare in rural communities. *Health & Social Care in the Community*, 10(4), 229–238.

Crisp, A. H., Gelder, M. G., Rix, S., Meltzer, H. I., & Rowlands, O. J. (2000). Stigmatisation of people with mental illnesses. *British Journal of Psychiatry*, 177, 4–7.

Cross, T., Bazron, B., Dennis, K., & Isaacs, M. (1989). *Toward a cultural competent system of care*. Washington, DC: Georgetown University.

Crozier, I. (2011). Making up koro: Multiplicity, psychiatry, culture, and penis-shrinking anxieties. *Journal of the History of Medicine and Allied Sciences*, 67, 36–70.

Cusack, J., Deane, F., Wilson, C., & Ciarrochi, J. (2004). Who influence men to go to therapy? Reports from men attending psychological services. *International Journal for the Advancement of Counselling*, 26(3), 271–283.

Davidson, L., Rakfeldt, J., & Strauss, J. S. (2010). *The roots of the recovery movement in psychiatry: Lessons learned*. London, England: Wiley-Blackwell.

Davis, L., Uezato, A., Newell, J. M., & Frazier, E. (2008). Major depression and comorbid substance use disorders. *Current Opinion in Psychiatry*, 21, 14–18.

De Geyndt, W. (1995). *Managing the quality of health care in developing countries*. World Bank Technical Paper, no. 258. Washington, D.C: World Bank.

Demyttenaere, K., Bruffaerts, R., Posada-Villa, Gasquet, I., Kovess, V., Lepine, J. P., …, WHO World Mental Health Survey Consortium (2004). Prevalence, severity, and unmet need for treatment of mental disorders in the World Health Organisation World Mental Health Surveys. *Journal of the American Medical Association*, 291(21), 2581–2590.

Department of Health. (2001). *National confidential inquiry into suicide and homicide by people with mental illness*. London: HMSO.

Department of Health. (2003). *Attitudes to mental illness*. London: DoH.

Department of Health. (2005). *Delivering race equality in mental health care: An action plan for reform inside and outside services and the government's response to the independent inquiry into the death of David Bennett*. London: DoH.

Department of Health and Human Services. (1999). *Mental health: A report of the Surgeon General*. Rockville, MD: U.S. Department of Health and Human Services.

Deressa, W., Ali, A., & Enqusellassie, F. (2003). Self-treatment of malaria in rural communities, Butajira, southern Ethiopia. *Bulletin of the World Health Organization*, 81, 261–268.

Desforges, D. M., Lord, C. G., Ramsey, S. L., Mason, J. A., Van Leeuwen, M. D., West, S. C., & Lepper, M. R. (1991). Effects of structured cooperative contact on changing negative attitudes toward stigmatized social groups. *Journal of Personality and Social Psychology*, 60, 531–544.

Dessoki, H. H., & Hifnawy, T. M. S. (2009). Beliefs about mental illness among university students in Egypt. *Europe's Journal of Psychology*, 5(1), 1–19.

Dietrich, S., Beck, M., Bujantugs, B., Kenzine, D., Matschinger, H., & Angermeyer, M. C. (2004). The relationship between public causal beliefs and social distance toward mentally ill people. *Australian and New Zealand Journal of Psychiatry*, 38(5), 348–354.

Dietrich, S., Heider, D., Matschinger, H., & Angermeyer, M. C. (2006). Influence of newspaper reporting on adolescents' attitudes toward people with mental illness. *Social Psychiatry and Psychiatric Epidemiology*, 41, 318–322.

Dinos, S., Ascoli, M., Owiti, J., & Bhui, K. (2017). Assessing explanatory models and health beliefs: An essential but overlooked competency for clinicians. *BJPsych Advances*, 23(2), 106–114.

Dinos, S., Stevens, S., Serfaty, M., Weich, S., & King, M. (2004). Stigma: The feelings and experiences of 46 people with mental illness. *British Journal of Psychiatry*, 184, 176–181.

Disability Discrimination Act. (2005). *A law to help disabled people*. London: HMSO.

Dixon, J. M. (2008). *Attitudes toward Acculturative Behavior Scale: Development, reliability and validity* (Doctoral thesis, Ohio University). Retrieved from https://etd.ohiolink.edu/!etd.send_file?accession=ohiou1210546951&disposition=inline.

Donati, F. (2000). Madness and morale: A chronic psychiatric ward. In R. Hinshelwood & W. Skogstad (Eds.). *Observing organisations* (pp. 29–43). London: Routledge.

Donnelly, L. P. (2005). Mental health beliefs and help seeking behavior of Korean American parents of adult children with schizophrenia. *The Journal of Multicultural Nursing & Health*, 11, 23–34.

Donnelly, P. J. (1992). The impact of culture on psychotherapy: Korean clients' expectations in psychotherapy. *The Journal of New York State Nurses Association*, 23(2), 12–15.

Doornbos, M. M., Zandee, G. L., DeGroot, J., & De Maagd-Rodriguez, M. (2013). Using community-based participatory research to explore social determinants of women's mental health and barriers to help-seeking in three urban, ethnically diverse, impoverished, and underserved communities. *Archives of Psychiatric Nursing*, 27(6), 278–284.

Dohrenwend, B. P. (1966). Social status and psychological disorder: An issue of substance and an issue of method. *American Sociological Review*, 31, 14–34.

Dosreis, S., Mychailyszyn, M. P., Evans-Lacko, S. E., Beltran, A., Riley, A. W., & Myers, M. A. (2009). The meaning of attention-deficit/hyperactivity disorder medication and parents' initiation and continuity of treatment for their child. *Journal of Child and Adolescent Psychopharmacology*, 19(4), 377–383.

Dow, H. D., & Woolley, S. R. (2011). Mental health perceptions and coping strategies of Albanian immigrants and their families. *Journal of Marital & Family Therapy*, 37(1), 95–108.

Drake, R. E., McHugo, G. J., Xie, H., Fox, M., Packard, J., & Helmstetter, B. (2006). Ten-year recovery outcomes for clients with co-occurring schizophrenia and substance use disorders. *Schizophrenia Bulletin*, 32, 464–473.

Drummond, P. D., Mizan, A., Brocx, K., & Wright, B. (2011). Barriers to accessing health care services for West African refugee women living in Western Australia. *Health Care for Women International*, 32(3), 206–224.

Druss, B. G., Marcus, S. C., Rosenheck, R. A., Olfson, M., Tanielian, T., & Pincus, H. A. (2000). Understanding disability in mental and general medical conditions. *American Journal of Psychiatry*, 157(9), 1485–1491.

Duckworth, K., Halpern, J. H., Schutt, R. K., & Gillespie, C. (2003). Use of schizophrenia as a metaphor in U.S. Newspapers. *Psychiatric Services*, 54, 1402–1404.

Dunn, S. (1991). *Mind Readings*. London: Mind.

Duxbury, J. (2002). An evaluation of staff and patient views of and strategies employed to manage inpatient aggression and violence on one mental health unit: a pluralistic design. *Journal of Psychiatric and Mental Health Nursing*, 9, 325–337.

Earle, K. A. (1998). Cultural diversity and mental health: The Haudenosaunee of New York State. *Social Work Research*, 22, 89–99.

Economou, M., Gramandani, C., Richardson, C., & Stefanis, C. (2005). Public attitudes towards people with schizophrenia in Greece. *World Psychiatry: Official Journal of the World Psychiatric Association (WPA)*, 4(1), 40–44.

Edelman, C. L., Kudzma, E., & Mandle, C. (2014). *Health Promotion throughout the Life Span*. St Louis: Mosby.

Edge, D., & Rogers, A. (2005). 'Dealing with it': Black Caribbean women's response to adversity and psychological distress associated with pregnancy, childbirth, and early motherhood. *Social Science and Medicine*, 61(1), 15–25.

Edwards, S. P., Grobbelaar, P. W., Sibaya, P. T., Nene, L. M., Kunene, S. T., & Magwaza, A. S. (1983). Traditional Zulu theories of illness in psychiatric patients. *The Journal of Social Psychology*, 121, 213–221.

El-Islam, M. F. (2000). Mental illness in Kuwait and Qatar. In I. Al-Issa (Ed.), *Al-Junun: Mental illness in the Islamic world* (pp. 121–137). Madison, CT: International Universities Press.

Elliot-Schmidt, R., & Strong, J. (1997). The concept of well-being in a rural setting: Understanding health and illness. *Australian Journal of Rural Health*, 5, 59–63.

Erickson, C. D., & al-Timimi, N. R. (2001). Providing mental health services to Arab Americans: Recommendations and considerations. *Cultural Diversity and Ethnic Minority Psychology*, 7, 308–327.

Eronen, M., Tihonen, J., & Hakola, P. (1996). Schizophrenia and homicidal behavior. *Schizophrenia Bulletin*, 22, 83–89.

Essandoh, P. K. (1995). Counseling issues with African college students. *The Counseling Psychologist*, 23, 348–360.

Esterberg, M. L., & Compton, M. T. (2006). Causes of schizophrenia reported by family members of urban African American hospitalized patients with schizophrenia. *Comprehensive Psychiatry*, 47, 221–226.

Evans-Lacko S. E., Baum, N., Danis, M., Biddle, A., & Goold, S. (2012). Laypersons' choices and deliberations for mental health coverage. *Administration and Policy in Mental Health*, 39(3), 158–169.

Evans-Lacko, S. E., Corker, E., Williams, P., Henderson, C., & Thornicraft, G. (2014). Effect of the Time to Change anti-stigma campaign on trends in mental-illness-related public stigma among the English population in 2003–13: An analysis of survey data. *The Lancet Psychiatry*, 1(2), 121–128.

Ewhrudjakpor, C. (2009). Knowledge, beliefs and attitude of health care providers towards the mentally ill in Delta State, Nigeria. *Studies on Ethno-Medicine*, 3(1), 19–25.

Ewhrudjakpor, C. (2010a). A comparative study of knowledge and attitude of urban and rural dwellers toward vagrant sufferers of schizophrenia in Delta State, Nigeria. *East African Journal of Public Health*, 7(2), 114–119.

Ewhrudjakpor, C. (2010b). Psychiatric institutions and the emerging institutional scene in Nigeria. *African Research Review*, 4(1), 132–147.

Fabiyi, O. (2013, October 15). Nigerians spend N250bn on medical tourism annually – Expert. *The Punch News online*. Retrieved from http://odili.net/news/source/2013/oct/16/816.html.

Fabrega, H. (1991). Psychiatric stigma in non-western societies. *Comprehensive Psychiatry*, 32, 534–551.

Falk, G. (2001). *Stigma: How we treat outsiders*. New York: Prometheus Books.

Fallot, R. (2001). Spirituality and religion in psychiatric rehabilitation. *International Review of Psychiatry*, 13, 110–116.

Farina, A. (1998). Stigma. In K. T. Mueser, & N. Tarrier (Eds.), *Handbook of social functioning in schizophrenia* (pp. 247–279). Boston: Allyn & Bacon.

Fazio, R. H. (1990). Multiple processes by which attitudes guide behavior – The mode model as an integrative framework. *Advances in Experimental Social Psychology*, 23, 74–109.

Federal Ministry of Health. (1991). *The National Mental Health Policy for Nigeria*. Abuja: Federal Ministry of Health.

Feldman, D. B., & Crandall, C. S. (2007). Dimensions of mental illness stigma: What about mental illness causes social rejection? *Journal of Social and Clinical Psychology*, 26, 137–154.

Festinger, L. (1957). *A theory of cognitive dissonance*. California: Stanford University Press.

Finzen, A. (1996). *Der Verwaltungsrat ist schizophren. Die Krankheit und das Stigma [The Board of Directors is schizophrenic. The disease and the stigma]*. Bonn, Germany: Psychiatrie-Verlag.

Fiske, S. T., & Taylor, S. E. (1991). *Social cognition*. London: McGraw-Hill, Inc.

Flaskerud, J. H. (1986). The effects of culture-compatible intervention on the utilization of mental health services by minority clients. *Community Mental Health Journal*, 22(2), 127–141.

Foskett, J., Marriott, J., & Wilson-Rudd, F. (2004). Mental health, religion and spirituality: Attitudes, experience and expertise among mental health professionals and religious leaders in Somerset. *Mental Health, Religion & Culture*, 7(1), 5–22.

Foster, R. P. (2001). When immigrant is trauma: Guideline for the individual and family clinician. *American Journal of Orthopsychiatry*, 71, 153–170.

Foucault, M. (1978). About the concept of the "dangerous individual" in 19th century legal psychiatry. *International Journal of Law and Psychiatry*, 1, 1–18.

Fox, J. C., Blank, M., Rovnyak, V. G., & Barnett, R. Y. (2001). Barriers to help seeking for mental disorders in a rural impoverished population. *Community Mental Health Journal*, 37(5), 421–436.

Francis, C., Pirkis, J., Dunt, D., & Blood, R. W. (2001). *Mental health and illness in the media: A review of the literature*. Canberra: Commonwealth Department of Health and Aged Care.

Freeman, M. (1992). *Providing mental health care for all in South Africa: Structure and strategy, Paper no. 4. Centre for the Study of Health Policy*. Johannesburg: Dept. of Community Health, Univerty of the Witwatersrand.

Freeman, M., & Motsei, M. (1992). Planning health care in South Africa: Is there a role for traditional healers? *Social Science and Medicine*, 35(11), 1183–1190.

Friedman, T., Newton, C., Coggan, C., Hooley, S., Patel, R., Pickard, M., & Mitchell, A. J. (2005). Predictors of A & E staff attitudes to self-harm patients who use self-laceration: Influence of previous training and experience. *Journal of Psychosomatic Research*, 60, 273–277.

Fujisawa, D., Hashimoto, N., Masamune-Koizumi, Y., Otsuka, K., Tateno, M., Okugawa, G., & Sartorius, N. (2008). Pathway to psychiatric care in Japan: A multicenter observational study. *International Journal of Mental Health Systems*, 2, 14.

Fuller, J., Edwards, J., Procter, N., & Moss, J. (2000). How definition of mental health problems can influence help seeking in rural and remote communities. *Australian Journal of Rural Health*, 8(3), 148–153.

Fung, K., & Wong, Y. L. (2007). Factors influencing attitudes toward seeking professional help among East and Southeast Asian immigrant and refugee women. *International Journal of Social Psychiatry*, 53, 216–231.

Furnham, A. (1997). Overcoming Neurosis: Lay attributions of cure for five specific disorders. *Journal of Clinical Psychology*, 53, 595–604.

Furnham, A., & Chan, E. (2004). Lay theories of schizophrenia. A cross-cultural comparison of British and Hong Kong Chinese attitudes, attributions and beliefs. *Social Psychiatry and Psychiatric Epidemiology*, 39, 543–552.

Furnham, A., & Igboaka, A. (2007). Young people's recognition and understanding of schizophrenia: A cross-cultural study of young people from Britain and Nigeria. *International Journal of Social Psychiatry*, 53(5), 430–446.

Gabbard, G. O., & Gabbard, K. (1992). Cinematic stereotypes contributing to the stigmatization of psychiatrists. In P. J. Fink and A. Tasman (Eds.), *Stigma and Mental Illness* (pp. 113–126). Washington DC: American Psychiatric Press.

Gaebel, W., Baumann, A., Witte, A. M., & Zaeske, H. (2002). Public attitudes towards people with mental illness in six German cities. *European Archives of Psychiatry and Clinical Neuroscience*, 252, 278–287.

Gaertner, S. L., Rust, M. C., Dovidio, J. F., Bachman, B. A., & Anastasio, P. A. (1996). The contact hypothesis: The role of a common in-group identity on reducing intergroup bias among majority and minority group members. In J. L. Nye, & A. M. Brower (Eds.), *What's social about social cognition?* (pp. 230–260). Thousand Oaks, CA: Sage.

Gafoor, M., & Rassool, H. G. (1998). The coexistence of psychiatric disorders and substance misuse: Working with dual diagnosis patients. *Journal of Advanced Nursing*, 27, 497–502.

Gaines, A. D. (1998). Mental illness and immigration. In S. Loue (Ed.), *Handbook of Immigrant Health* (pp. 407–422). New York: Plenum.

Gale, E. (2001). Promoting promotion. *Openmind*, 110, 14–15.

Galli, U., Ettlin, D. A., Palla, S., Ehlert, U., & Gaab, J. (2010). Do illness perceptions predict pain-related disability and mood in chronic orofacial pain patients? A 6-month follow-up study. *European Journal of Pain*, 14, 550–558.

García-Moreno, C. (2002). Dilemas and opportunities for an appropriate health-service response to violence against women. *Lancet*, 359, 1509–1514.

Garfield, R. L., Zuvekas, S. H., Lave, J. R., & Donohue, J. M. (2011). The impact of national health care reform on adults with severe mental disorders. *American Journal of Psychiatry*, 168, 486–494.

Gash, H., & Coffey, D. (1995). Influences on attitudes towards children with mental handicap. *European Journal of Special Needs Education*, 10, 1–16.

Gater, R., De Almeida E., Sousa, B., Barrientos, G., Caraveo, J., Chandrashekar, C. R., ... Silhan, K. (1991). The pathways to psychiatric care: A cross-cultural study. *Psychological Medicine*, 21, 761–774.

Gater, R., Jordanova, V., Maric, N., & Alikaj, V. (2005). Pathways to psychiatric care in Eastern Europe. *British ournal of Psychiatry*, 186, 529–535.

GBD 2017 Disease and Injury Incidence and Prevalence Collaborators. (2018). Global health metrics. *Lancet*, 392, 1789–1858.

Gehlot, P. S., & Nathawat, S. S. (1983). Suicide and family constellation in India. *British Journal of Psychotherapy*, 37, 273–278.

Geller, J. M. 1999. Rural primary care providers' perceptions of their roles in the provision of mental health services: Voices from the plains. *Journal of Rural Health*, 15(3), 326–334.

Gellis, Z. D., Huh, N. S., Lee, S., & Kim, J. (2003). Mental health attitudes among Caucasian-American and Korean counseling students. *Community Mental Health Journal*, 39(3), 213–224.

Gerace, L. M., Hughes, T. L., & Spunt, J. (1995). Improving nurses' responses toward substance-misusing patients: A clinical evaluation project. *Archives of Psychiatric Nursing*, 9, 286–294.

Gilbert, P., Gilbert, J., & Sanghera, J. (2004). A focus group exploration of the impact of izzat, shame, subordination and entrapment on mental health service use in South Asian Women living in Derby. *Mental Health, Religion and Culture*, 7, 109–130.

Gilbert, P., Bhundia, R., Mitra, R., McEwan, K., Irons, C., & Sanghera, J. (2007). Cultural differences in shame-focused attitudes towards mental health problems in Asian and Non-Asian student women. *Mental Health, Religion & Culture*, 10(2), 127–141.

Gillborn, D., & Gibbs, C. (1996). *Recent research on the achievement of ethnic minority pupils*. London: HMSO.

Girma, E., & Tesfaye, M. (2011). Patterns of treatment seeking behavior for mental illness in Southwest Ethiopia: A hospital based study. *BMC Psychiatry*, 11, 138.

Goetz, E. R., Camargo, B. V., Bertoldo, R. B., & Justo, A. M. (2008). Representação social do corpo na mídia impressa. *Psicologia e Sociedade*, 20(2), 226–236.

Goffman, E. (1967). *Interaction rituals: Essays in face-to-face behaviour*. Chicago, IL: Aldine.

Good, G. E., & Wood, K. (1995). Male gender role conflict, depression, and help seeking: Do college men face double jeopardy? *Journal of Counseling & Development*, 74, 70–75.

Goodman, D. (1992). Link of violent crime to mentally illness dispelled by researcher. *Public Health Reports*, 107(1), 126–128.

Gournay, K. (1996). Double bind. *Nursing Times*, 92, 28–29.

Graham, N., Lindesay, J., Katona, C., Bertolote, J. M., Camus, V., Copeland, J. R. M., ... World Health Organization (2003). Reducing stigma and discrimination against older people with mental disorders: A technical consensus statement. *International Journal of Geriatric Psychiatry*, 18, 670–678.

Granerud, A., & Severinsson, E. (2006). The struggle for social integration in the community – the experiences of people with mental health problems. *Journal of Psychiatric and Mental Health Nursing*, 13(3), 288–293.

Grausgruber, A., Meise, U., Katschnig, H., Schöny, W., & Fleischhacker, W. W. (2007). Patterns of social distance towards people suffering from schizophrenia in Austria: A comparison between the general public, relatives and mental health staff. *Acta Psychiatrica Scandinavica*, 115(4), 310–319.

Gray, A. J. (2001). Attitudes of the public to mental health: A church congregation. *Mental Health, Religion & Culture*, 4(1), 71–79.

Green, G., Hayes, C., Dickinson, D., Whitaker, A., & Gilheaney, B. (2003). A mental health service users perspective to stigmatisation. *Journal of Mental Health*, 12, 223–234.

Griffiths, K. M., Nakane, Y., Christensen, H., Yoshioka, K., Jorm, A. F., & Nakane, H. (2006). Stigma in response to mental disorders: a comparison of Australia and Japan. *BMC Psychiatry*, 6, 21.

Griffiths, R., & Pearson, B. (1988). *Working with Drug Users*. Hampshire: Wildwood House.

Guerra, N. G., & Jagers, R. (1998). The importance of culture in the assessment of children and youth. In V. C. McLoyd & L. Steinberg (Eds.), *Studying minority adolescents: Conceptual, methodological, and theoretical issues* (pp. 123–142). Mahwah, NJ: Erlbaum.

Gulbinat, W., Manderscheid, R., Baingana, F., Jenkins, R., Khandelwal, S., Levav, I., ... Whiteford, H. (2004). The International Consortium on Mental Health Policy and Services: Objectives, design and project implementation. *International Review of Psychiatry*, 16(1–2), 5–17.

Gulliver, A., Griffiths, K. M., & Christensen, H. (2010). Perceived barriers and facilitators to mental health help-seeking in young people: A systematic review. *BMC Psychiatry*, 10, 113.

Gureje, O. (2003). Country profile: Psychiatry in Nigeria. *International Psychiatry*, 2, 10–12.

Gureje, O. (2007). Psychiatry in Africa: The myths, the exotic, and the realities. *South African Psychiatric Review*, 10, 11–14.

Gureje, O., Abdulmalik, J., Kola, L., Musa, E., Yasamy, M. T., & Adebayo, K. (2015). Integrating mental health into primary care in Nigeria: Report of a demonstration project using the mental health gap action programme intervention guide. *BMC Health Services Research*, 15, 242.

Gureje, O., & Alem, A. (2000). Mental health policy development in Africa. *Bulletin of World Health Organisation*, 78(4), 475–482.

Gureje, O., Acha, R. A., & Odejide, O. A. (1995). Pathways to psychiatric care in Ibadan. Nigeria. *Tropical and Geographical Medicine*, 47(3), 125–129.

Gureje, O., & Bamidele, R. (1999). Thirteen-year social outcome among Nigerian outpatients with schizophrenia. *Social Psychiatry and Psychiatric Epidemiology*, 34(3), 147–151.

Gureje, O., & Lasebikan, V. O. (2006). Use of mental health services in a developing country: Results from the Nigerian survey of mental health and well-being. *Social Psychiatry and Psychiatric Epidemiology*, 41(1), 44–49.

Gureje, O., Olley, O. O., Ephraim-Oluwanuga, O., & Kola, L. (2006). Do beliefs about causation influence attitudes to mental illness. *World Psychiatry: Official Journal of the World Psychiatric Association (WPA)*, 5, 104–107.

Gureje, O., Lasebikan, V. O., Ephraim-Oluwanuga, O., Olley, B. O., & Kola, L. (2005). Community study of knowledge of and attitude to mental illness in Nigeria. *British Journal of Psychiatry*, 186, 436–441.

Gutierrez-Lobos, K. (2002). Rechtliche Benachteiligung psychisch Kranker in bsterreich. (Legal discrimination of mentally disordered persons in Austria). *J Neuropsychiatrie*, 16, 22–26.

Haghighat, R. (2001). A unitary theory of stigmatisation: Pursuit of self interest and routes to destigmatisation. *British Journal of Psychiatry*, 178, 207–215.

Hall, L., & Tucker, C. (1985). Relationships between ethnicity, conceptions of mental illness, and attitudes associated with seeking psychological help. *Psychological Reports*, 57, 907–916.

Halm, E. A., Mora, P., & Leventhal, H. (2006). No symptoms, no asthma. The acute episodic disease belief is associated with poor self-management among inner-city adults with persistent asthma. *Chest*, 129, 573–580.

Hamid, P. D., Simmonds, J. G., & Bowles, T. V. (2009). Asian Australian acculturation and attitudes toward seeking professional psychological help. *Australian Journal of Psychology*, 61, 69–76.

Hannigan, B. (1999). Mental healthcare in the community: An analysis of contemporary public attitudes towards, and public representations of, mental illness. *Journal of Mental Health*, 8(5), 431–440.

Hansson, L., Jorrnfeldt, H., Svedberg, P., & Svensson, B. (2013). Mental health professionals' attitudes towards people with mental illness. Do they differ from attitudes held by people with mental illness? *International Journal of Social Psychiatry*, 59, 48–54.

Hagger, M. S., & Orbell, S. (2003). A meta-analytic review of the common-sense model of illness representations. *Psychology and Health*, 18, 141–184.

Harrison, G., Hopper, K., Craig, T., Laska, E., Siegel, C., Wanderling, J., ... Wiersma, D. (2001). Recovery from psychotic illness: A 15- and 25-year international follow-up study. *British Journal of Psychiatry*, 178, 506–517.

Harrison, M., Koenig, H., Hays, J., Eme-Akwari, A., & Pargament, K. (2001). The epidemiology of religious coping: A review of recent literature. *International Review of Psychiatry*, 13, 86–93.

Hartley, D., Korsea, N., Bird, D., & Agger, M. (1998). Management of patients with depression by rural primary care practitioners. *Archives of Family Medicine*, 7, 139–145.

Hawton, K., Daniels, R., & James, R. (1995). General Hospital services for attempted suicide patients: A survey in one region. *Health Trends*, 27, 18–21.

Hemmens, C., Miller, M., Burton, V. S., & Milner, S. (2002). The consequences of official labels: An examination of the rights lost by the mentally ill and mentally incompetent ten years later. *Community Mental Health*, 38, 129–140.

Henderson, C., Corker, E., Lewis-Holmes, E., Hamilton, S., Flach, C., Rose, D., ... Thornicroft, G. (2012). Reducing mental health related stigma and discrimination in England: One year outcomes of the Time to Change Programme for service user-rated experiences of discrimination. *Psychiatric Services*, 63(5), 451–457.

Hitchens, D. (2015). The remarkable case of Mr B. *The Catholic Herald*, 24, 6732.

Hines-Martin, V., Brown-Piper, A., Kim, S., & Malone, M. (2003). Enabling factors of mental health service use among African Americans. *Archives of Psychiatric Nursing*, 17(5), 197–204.

Hinshaw, S. P., & Stier, A. (2008). Stigma as related to mental disorders. *Annual Review of Clinincal Psychology*, 4, 367–393.

Högberg, T., Magnusson, A., Ewertzon, M., & Lützén, K. (2008). Attitudes towards mental illness in Sweden: Adaptation and development of the community attitudes towards mental illness questionnaire. *International Journal of Mental Health Nursing*, 17, 302–310.

Hoge, C. W., Castro, C. A., Messer, S. C., McGurk, D., Cotting, D. I., & Koffman, R. L. (2004). Combat duty in Iraq and Afghanistan, mental health problems, and barriers to care. *New England Journal of Medicine*, 351(1), 13–22.

Hopper, K., & Wanderling, J. (2000). Revisiting the developed versus developing country distinction in course and outcome in schizophrenia: Results from ISoS, the WHO collaborative follow-up project. *Schizophrenia Bulletib*, 26(4), 835–846.

Hough, R. L., Willging, C. E., Altschul, D., & Adelsheim, S. (2011). Workforce capacity for reducing rural disparities in public mental health services for adults with severe mental illness. *Rural Mental Health*, 35(2), 35–45.

Howerton, A., Byng, R., Campbell, J., Hess, D., Owens, C., & Aitken, P. (2007). Understanding help-seeking behaviour among male offenders: Qualitative interview study. *British Medical Journal*, 334(7588), 303.

Hsu, G. (2003). *Priorities for Asian American mental health*. Paper presented at the Conference of the NY Coalition for Asian American Mental Health on Beyond Cultural Competence: Challenges and opportunities for Asian American Mental Health, New York.

Hugo, M. (2001). Mental health professionals' attitudes towards people who have experienced a mental health disorder. *Journal of Psychiatric Mental Health Nursing*, 8(5), 419–425.

Hugo, C. J., Boshoff, D. E., Traut, A., Zungu-Dirwayi, N., & Stein, D. J. (2003). Community attitudes toward and knowledge of mental illness in South Africa. *Social Psychiatry and Psychiatry Epidemiology*, 38, 715–719.

Hundertmark, J. (2002). The impact of mainstreaming on patient care in Australian Emergency Departments and liaison services. *Australian and New Zealand Journal of Psychiatry*, 36, 424.

Hunter, L. R., & Schmidt, N. B. (2010). Anxiety psychopathology in African American adults: Literature review and development of an empirically informed sociocultural model. *Psychological Bulletin*, 136(2), 211–235.

Huxley, P. (1993). Location and stigma: A survey of community attitudes to mental illness. *Journal of Mental Health*, 2, 73–80.

Hwang, W. C., Myers, H. F., Abe-Kim, J., & Ting, J. Y. (2008). A Conceptual Paradigm for understanding culture's impact on mental health: The cultural influences on mental health (CIMH) model. *Clinical Psychology Review*, 28(2), 211–227.

Idemudia, E. S. (2004). Mental Health and Psychotherapy through the eyes of culture: Lessons for African Psychotherapy. In H. Arlt and E. S. Idemudia (Eds.), *The unifying aspects of cultures* (pp. 230–232). Vienna, Austria.

Ogunmade, O. (2013, June 5). NACA: Nigeria is second largest carrier of HIV/AIDS. *Thisday Newspaper.* Retrieved from http://www.thisdaylive.com/articles/naca-nigeria-is-second-largest-carrier-of-hiv-aids-in-the-world/149428/.

Igbinomwanhia, N. G., James, B. O., & Omoaregba, J. O. (2013). The attitudes of clergy in Benin City, Nigeria towards persons with mental illness. *African Journal of Psychiatry*, 16, 196–200.

Ikwuka, U., Galbraith, N., & Nyatanga, L. (2014). Causal attribution of mental illness in south-eastern Nigeria. *International Journal of Social Psychiatry*, 60(3), 274–279.

Ikwuka, U. (2016). *Perceptions of mental illness in south-eastern Nigeria: Causal beliefs, attitudes, help-seeking pathways and perceived barriers to help-seeking.* (Doctoral thesis, University of Wolverhampton, UK). Retrieved from https://ethos.bl.uk/OrderDetails.do?uin=uk.bl.ethos.767205.

Jablensky, A., Sartorius, N., Ernberg, G., Anker, M., Korten, A., Cooper, J. E., ... Bertelsen, A. (1992). Schizophrenia: manifestations, incidence and course in different cultures: A World Health Organization ten-country study. *Psychological Medicine, Monograph Supplement*, 20, 1–97.

Jack-Ide, I. O., Makoro, B. P., & Azibiri, B. (2013). Pathways to mental health care services in the Niger Delta region of Nigeria. *Journal of Research in Nursing and Midwifery*, 2(2), 22–29.

Jack-Ide, I. O., & Uys, L. (2013). Barriers to mental health services utilization in the Niger Delta region of Nigeria: Service users' perspectives. *Pan African Medical Journal*, 14, 159.

Jack-Ide, I. O., Uys, L., & Middleton, L. E. (2013). Caregiving experiences of families of persons with serious mental health problems in the Niger Delta region of Nigeria. *International Journal of Mental Health Nursing*, 22(2), 170–179.

Jagdeo, A., Cox, B. J., Stein, M. B., & Sareen, J. (2009). Negative attitudes toward help seeking for mental illness in 2 population-based surveys from the United States and Canada. *Canadian Journal of Psychiatry*, 54(11), 757–766.

Jang, Y., Kim, G., Hansen, L., & Chiriboga, D. L. (2007). Attitudes of older Korean Americans toward mental health services. *Journal of American Geriatrics Society*, 55(4), 616–620.

Jelen, T. G. (1984). Respect for life, sexual morality, and opposition to abortion. *Review of Religious Research*, 25, 220–231.

Jenkins, J. H., & Karno, M. (1992). The meaning of expressed emotion: Theoretical issues raised by cross-cultural research. *American Journal of Psychiatry*, 149(1), 9–21.

Johannessen, J. O., McGlashan, T. H., Larsen, T. K., Horneland, M., Joa, I., Mardal, S., ... Vaglum, P. (2001). Early detection strategies for untreated first-episode psychosis. *Schizophrenia Research*, 51(1), 39–46.

Jones, E. E., Farina, A., Hastorf, A. H., Marcus, H., Miller, D. T., & Scott, R. A. (1984). *Social stigma: The psychology of marked relationships.* New York: Freeman and Company.

Jorm, A. F. (2000). Mental health literacy: Public knowledge and beliefs about mental disorders. *British Journal of Psychiatry*, 177, 396–401.

Jorm, A. F., & Griffiths, K. M. (2008). The public's stigmatizing attitudes towards people with mental disorders: How important are biomedical conceptualizations? *Acta Psychiatrica Scandinavica*, 118(4), 315–321.

Jorm, A. F., Korten, A. E., Jacomb, P. A., Christensen, H., Rodgers, B., & Pollitt, P. (1997). "Mental health literacy": A survey of the public's ability to recognise mental disorders and their beliefs about the effectiveness of treatment. *Medical Journal of Australia*, 166, 182–186.

Jorm, A. F., Korten, A. E., Jacomb, P. A., Rodgers, B., & Pollitt, P. (1997). Helpfulness of interventions for mental disorders: Beliefs of health professionals compared with the general public. *British Journal of Psychiatry*, 171, 233–237.

Jorm, A., & Oh, E. (2009). Desire for social distance from people with mental disorders: A review. *Australian and New Zealand Journal of Psychiatry*, 43, 183–200.

Judd, F., Komiti, A., & Jackson, H. (2008). How does being female assist help-seeking for mental health problems? *Australian and New Zealand Journal of Psychiatry*, 42, 24–29.

Kabir, M., Iliyasu, Z., Abubakar, I. S., & Aliyu, M. H. (2004). Perception and beliefs about mental illness among adults in Karfi village, northern Nigeria. *BMC International Health and Human Rights*, 4(1), 3.

Kadri, N., Manoudi, F., Berrada, S., & Moussaoui, D. (2004). Stigma impact on Moroccan families of patients with schizophrenia. *Canadian Journal of Psychiatry*, 49(9), 625–629.

Kamya, H. A. (2001). African immigrants in the United States: The challenge for research and practice. *Social Work*, 42(2), 154–165.

Kaptein, A. A., Bijsterbosch, J., Scharloo, M., Hampson, S. E., Kroon, H. M., & Kloppenburg, M. (2010). Using the common sense model of illness perceptions to examine osteoarthritis change: A 6-year longitudinal study. *Health Psychology*, 29, 56–64.

Kassam, N. (1997). *Telling it like it is: Young Asian women talk*. London: Livewire/Women's Press.

Katung, P. Y. (2001). Socio-economic factors responsible for poor utilisation of the primary health care services in a rural community in Nigeria. *Nigerian Journal of Medicine*, 10(1), 28–29.

Kate, N., Grover, S., Kulhara, P., & Nehra, R. (2012). Supernatural beliefs, aetiological models and help seeking behaviour in patients with schizophrenia. *Industrial Psychiatry Journal*, 21(1), 49–54.

Keane, M. (1991). Acceptance vs. rejection: Nursing students' attitudes about mental illness. *Perspectives in Psychiatric Care*, 27(3), 13–18.

Keating, F., Robertson, D., McCulloch, A., & Francis, E. (2002). *Breaking the circles of fear: A review of the relationship between mental health services and African and Caribbean communities*. London: The Sainsbury Centre for Mental Health.

Keating F., & Robertson, D. (2004). Fear, black people and mental illness: A vicious circle? *Health and Social Care in the Community*, 12(5), 439–447.

Kelly, C., Jorm, A., & Wright, A. (2007). Improving mental health literacy as a strategy to facilitate early intervention for mental disorders. *Medical Journal of Australia*, 187(7), 26–30.

Kemali, D., Maj, M., Veltro, F., Crepet, P., & Lobrace, S. (1989). Sondaggio sulle opinioni degli italiani nei riguardi dei malati di mente e della situazione dell'assistenza psichiatrica. *Rivista Sperimentale di Freniatria*, 5, 1301–1351.

Kermode, M., Bowen, K., Arole, S., Pathare, S., & Jorm, A. F. (2009). Attitudes to people with mental disorders: A mental health literacy survey in a rural area of Maharashtra, India. *Social Psychiatry and Psychiatric Epidemiology*, 44(12), 1087–1096.

Kessler, R. C., Berglund, P. A., Bruce, M. L., Koch, J. R., Laska, E. M., Leaf, P. J., ... Wang, P. S. (2001). The prevalence and correlates of untreated serious mental illness. *Health Services Research*, 36(6), 987–1007.

Keusch, G. T., Wilentz, J., & Kleinman, A. (2006). Stigma and global health: Developing a research agenda. *Lancet*, 367, 525–527.

Keynejad, R. (2008). *Barriers to seeking help: What stops ethnic minority groups in Redbridge accessing mental health services?* Essex: Redbridge CVS.

Khandelwal, S. K., & Workneh, F. (1986). Perception of mental illness by medical students. *Indian Journal of Psychological Medicine*, 9, 26–32.

Khoweiled, A. (2005). Attitude of a sample of Egyptian General Practitioners and newly graduated medical students towards psychiatric illness. *The Egyptian Journal of Mental Health*, 42, 1–29.

Kiger, G. (1992). Disability simulations: Logical, methodological and ethical issues. *Disability, Handicap & Society*, 7, 71–78.

King, P., Judd, F., & Grigg, M. (2001). *A model for consultation liaison psychiatry in the Loddon Southern Mallee Region for Victoria Project Report*. Bendigo: Bendigo Health Care Group Psychiatric Services.

Kingdon, D., Sharma, T., Hart, D. (2004). The Schizophrenia subgroup of the Royal College of Psychiatrists' Changing Minds Campaign. What attitudes do psychiatrists hold towards people with mental illness? *Psychiatric Bulletin* 28, 401–406.

Kirmayer, L. J., Groleau, D., Looper, K. J., & Dominicé, M. (2004). Explaining medically unexplained symptoms. *The Canadian Journal of Psychiatry/LaRevue Canadienne De Psychiatrie*, 49(10), 663–672.

Kirmayer, L. J., & Jarvis, G. E. (2006). Depression across cultures. In D. J. Stein, A. F. Schatzberg, & D. J. Kupfer (Eds.), *The American Psychiatric Publishing textbook of mood disorders* (pp. 699–715). Washington, DC: American Psychiatric Association Press.

Kitchener, B. A., & Jorm, A. F. (2002). Mental health first aid training for the public: Evaluation of effects on knowledge, attitudes and helping behavior. *BMC Psychiatry*, 2, 10.

Kleinman, A. M. (1977). Depression, somatization and the 'new cross-cultural psychiatry'. *Social Science and Medicine*, 11, 3–10.

Kleinman, A. M. (1980). *Patients and healers in the context of culture: An exploration of the borderland between anthropology, medicine, and psychiatry*. Berkeley: University of California Press.

Kleinman, A. M. (1987). Anthropology and psychiatry: The role of culture in cross-cultural research on illness. *British Journal of Psychiatry*, 151, 447–454.

Kleinman, A. M. (2009). Global mental health: A failure of humanity. *Lancet*, 374, 603–604.

Kleintjes, S., Lund, C., & Flisher, A. J. (2010). MHAPP Research Programme Consortium. A situational analysis of child and adolescent mental health services in Ghana, Uganda, South Africa and Zambia. *African Journal of Psychiatry*, 13, 132–139.

Kobau, R., DiIorio, C., Chapman, D., & Delvecchio, P. (2010). Attitudes about mental illness and its treatment: Validation of a Generic Scale for public health surveillance of mental illness associated stigma. *Community Mental Health Journal*, 46, 164–176.

Koenig, H. G. (2008). Religion and mental health: What should psychiatrists do? *Psychiatrist*, 32, 201–203.

Komiti, A., Judd, F., & Jackson, H. (2006). The influence of stigma and attitudes on seeking help from a GP for mental health problems: A rural context. *Social Psychiatry and Psychiatric Epidemiology*, 41, 738–745.

Krauss, S. J. (1995). Attitudes and the prediction of behavior: A metaanalysis of the empirical literature. *Personality and Social Psychology Bulletin*, 21, 58–75.

Kunda, Z., & Oleson, K. C. (1995). Maintaining stereotypes in the face of disconfirmation: Constructing grounds for subtyping deviants. *Journal of Personality and Social Psychology*, 68, 565–579.

Kung, W. W. (2003). The illness, stigma, culture, or immigration? Burdens on Chinese American caregivers of patients with schizophrenia. *Families in Society*, 84(4), 547–557.

Kurihara, T., Kato, M., Reverger, R., & Tirta, I. (2006). Beliefs about causes of schizophrenia among family members: A community-based survey in Bali. *Psychiatric Services*, 57, 1795–1799.

Kushner, M. G., & Sher, K. J. (1991). The relation of treatment fearfulness and psychological services utilization: An overview. *Professional Psychology: Research and Practice*, 22, 196–203.

Lahariya, C., Singhai, S., Gupta, S., & Mishra, A. (2010). Pathway of care among psychiatric patients attending a mental health institution in central India. *Indian Journal of Psychiatry*, 52(4), 333–338.

Lam, C. S., Tsang, H., Chan, F., & Corrigan, P. W. (2006). Chinese and American perspectives on stigma. *Rehabilitation Education*, 20, 269–279.

Lambo, T. A. (1978). Psychotherapy in Africa. *Human Nature*, 1(3), 32–39.

Lalani, N., & London, C. (2006). 'The media: Agents of social exclusion for people?' Politics of Health Group. *UK Health Watch*, 99, 1–5.

Larson, J. E., & Corrigan, P. (2008). The stigma of families with mental illness. *Academic Psychiatry*, 32, 87–91.

Lauber, C., & Rössler, W. (2007). Stigma towards people with mental illness in developing countries in Asia. *International Review of Psychiatry*, 19, 157–178.

Lauria-Horner, B. A., Kutcher, S., & Brooks, S. J. (2004). The feasibility of a mental health curriculum in elementary school. *Canadian Journal of Psychiatry*, 49, 208–211.

Lawani, A. O. (2008). *The Nigerian society as a psychiatric patient*. Paper presented at the Annual Scientific Conference and workshop of Nigerian Association of Clinical Psychologists. Benin City, Nigeria.

Leaf, P. J., Livingston, M., & Tischler, G. L. (1986). The differential effect of attitudes on the use of mental health services. *Social Psychiatry*, 21, 187–192.

Lecrubier, Y. (2005). Posttraumatic stress disorder in primary care: A hidden diagnosis. *Journal of Clinical Psychiatry*, 65, 49–54.

Leff, J., & Warner, R. (2006). *Social inclusion of people with mental illness.* Cambridge: Cambridge University Press.

Le Meyer, O., Zane, N., Cho, Y. I., & Takeuchi, D. T. (2009). Use of specialty mental health services by Asian Americans with psychiatric disorders. *Journal of Consulting and Clinical Psychology*, 77(5), 1000–1005.

Leininger, M., & McFarland, M. R. (2002). *Transcultural Nursing: Concepts, theories, research and practice.* New York: McGraw Hill Co.

Leong, F., & Lau, A. (2001). Barriers to providing effective mental health services to Asian Americans. *Mental Health Services Research*, 3, 201–214.

Levav, I., Shemesh, A., Grinshpoon, A., Aisenberg, E., Shershevsky, Y., & Kohn, R. (2004). Mental health-related knowledge, attitudes and practices in two kibbutzim. *Social Psychiatry and Psychiatric Epidemiology*, 39, 758–764.

Levey, S., & Howells, K. (1994). Accounting for the fear of schizophrenia. *Journal of Community & Applied Social Psychology*, 4, 313–328.

Levey, S., & Howells, K. (1995). Dangerousness, unpredictability and the fear of people with schizophrenia. *Journal of Forensic Psychiatry*, 6, 19–39.

Liang, B., Goodman, L., Tummala-Narra, P., & Weintraub, S. (2005). A theoretical framework for understanding help-seeking processes among survivors of intimate partner violence. *American Journal of Community Psychology*, 36, 71–84.

Liberman, R. P. (2008). *Recovery from disability: Manual of psychiatric rehabilitation.* Washington, DC: American Psychiatric Publishing.

Liggins, J., & Hatcher, S. (2005). Stigma toward the mentally ill in the general hospital: A qualitative study. *General Hospital Psychiatry*, 27, 359–364.

Lin, K. M., Inui, T. S., Kleinman, A. M., & Womack, W. M. (1982). Sociocultural determinants of the help-seeking behavior of patients with mental illness. *Journal of Nervous and Mental Disease*, 170(2), 78–85.

Lincoln, C. V., & McGorry, P. (1995). Who cares? Pathways to psychiatric care for young people experiencing a first episode of psychosis. *Psychiatric Services*, 46, 1166–1171.

Lindisfarne, N. (1998). Gender, shame and culture: An anthropological perspective. In P. Gilbert & B. Andrews (Eds.), *Shame: Interpersonal behaviour, psychopathology and culture* (pp. 246–260). New York: Oxford University Press.

Link, B. G. (1982). Mental patient status, work, and income: An examination of the effects of a psychiatric label. *American Sociological Review*, 47, 202–215.

Link, B. G., Cullen, F. T., Struening, E. L., Shrout, P. E., & Dohrenwend, B. P. (1989). A modified labeling theory approach to mental disorders: An empirical assessment. *American Sociological Review*, 54, 400–423.

Link, B. G., Mirotznik, J., & Cullen, F. T. (1991). The effectiveness of stigma coping orientations: Can negative consequences of mental illness labeling be avoided? *Journal of Health and Social Behavior*, 32, 302–320.

Link, B. G., & Phelan, J. C. (2001). Conceptualizing stigma. *Annual Review of Sociology*, 27, 363–385.

Link, B. G., & Phelan, J. C. (2006). Stigma and its public health implications. *Lancet*, 367, 528–529.

Link, B. G., Phelan, J. C., Bresnahan, M., Stueve, A., & Pescosolido, B. A. (1999). Public conceptions of mental illness: Labels, causes, dangerousness, and social distance. *American Journal of Public Health*, 89, 1328–1333.

Link, B. G., Struening, E. L., Neese-Todd, S., Asmussen, A., & Phelan, J. C. (2001). Stigma as a barrier to recovery: The consequences of stigma for the self-esteem of people with mental illnesses. *Psychiatric Services*, 52, 1621–1626.

Link, B. G., Struening, E. L., Rahav, M., Phelan, J. C., & Nuttbrock, L. (1997). On stigma and its consequences: Evidence from a longitudinal study of men with dual diagnosis of mental illness and substance abuse. *Journal of Health and Social Behaviour*, 38, 177–190.

Link, B. G., Yang, L. H., Phelan, J. C., & Collins, P. Y. (2004). Measuring mental illness stigma. *Schizophrenia Bulletin*, 30, 511–541.

Littlewood, R. (1996). Psychiatry's culture. *International Journal of Social Psychiatry*, 42(4), 245–268.

Litwak, E. (1968). Technological innovation and theoretical functions of primary groups and bureaucratic structures. *American Journal of Sociology*, 73, 468–481.

Livaditis, M. (1994). *Psychiatry and the Law*. Athens Greece: Papazissis.

Lowe, T., Bond, K., Spokes, K., & Wellman, N. (2002). HOVIS – The Hertfordshire and Oxfordshire Violent Incident Study. *Journal of Psychiatric and Mental Health Nursing*, 9(2), 199–211.

Lucksted, A., & Drapalski, A. L. (2015). Self-stigma regarding mental illness: Definition, impact, and relationship to societal stigma. *Psychiatric Rehabilitation Journal*, 38(2), 99–102.

Maccoby, E. E. (1990). Gender and relationship: A development account. *American Psychologist*, 45, 513–420.

Mackenzie, C. S., Gekoski, W. L., & Knox, V. J. (2006). Age, gender, and the underutilization of mental health services: The influence of help-seeking attitudes. *Aging & Mental Health*, 10(6), 574–582.

MacLachlan, M. (1997). *Culture and health*. Chichester, UK: Wiley.

Magliano, L., Fiorillo, A., de Rosa, C., Malangone, C., & Maj, M. (2004). Beliefs about schizophrenia in Italy: A comparative nationwide survey of the general public, mental health professionals, and patients' relatives. *Canadian Journal of Psychiatry*, 49, 322–330.

Magliano, L., Fiorillo, A., de Rosa, C., Malangone, C., & Maj, M. (2005). Family burden in long-term diseases: A comparative study in schizophrenia vs. physical disorders. *Social Science & Medicine*, 61, 313–322.

Makanjuola, V. Y., Esan, B., Oladeji, Kola, L., Appiah-Poku, J., Harris, B., ... Gureje, O. (2016). Explanatory model of psychosis: Impact on perception of self-stigma by patients in three sub-saharan African cities. *Social Psychiatry & Psychiatric Epidemiology*, 51(12), 1645–1654.

Marcussen, K., Gallagher, M., & Ritter, C. (2018). Mental illness as a stigmatized identity. *Society and Mental Health*, 9(2), 211–227.

Marie, D., & Miles, B. (2008). Social distance and perceived dangerousness across four diagnostic categories of mental disorder. *Australian and New Zealand Journal of Psychiatry*, 42, 126–133.

Markowitz, F. E. (2014). Labeling theory and mental illness. In D. P. Farrington & J. Murray (Eds.), *Labeling theory: Empirical tests* (pp. 45–62). New Brunswick, NJ: Transaction.

Martin, J. K., Pescosolido, B. A., Olafsdottir, S., & McLeod, J. D. (2007). The construction of fear: Americans' preferences for social distance from children and adolescents with mental health problems. *Journal of Health and Social Behaviour*, 48, 50–67.

Martin, S. (2009). Illness of the mind or illness of the spirit? Mental health-related conceptualization and practices of older Iranian immigrants. *Health & Social Work*, 34, 117–126.

Mathers, C. D., Loncar, D. (2006). Projections of global mortality and burden of disease from 2002-2030. *PLoS Medicine*, 3(11), e442.

Maughan, B. (2005). Educational attainments: Ethnic differences in the United Kingdom. In M. Rutter & M. Tienda (Eds.), *Ethnicity and Causal Mechanisms* (pp. 80–106). New York: Cambridge University Press.

McCombie, S. C. (2002). Self-treatment for malaria: The evidence and methodological issues. *Health Policy and Planning*, 17, 333–344.

McConachie, S., & Whitford, H. (2009). Mental health nurses' attitudes towards severe perinatal mental illness. *Journal of Advanced Nursing*, 65(4), 867–876.

Mechanic, D. (1968). *Medical sociology: A selective view*. New York: The Free Press.

Mehta, N., Kassam, A., Leese, M., Butler, G., & Thornicroft, G. (2009). Public attitudes towards people with mental illness in England and Scotland, 1994-2003. *British Journal of Psychiatry*, 194(3), 278–284.

Meltzer, H., Bebbington, P. E., Brugha, T. S., Farrell, M., Jenkins, R., & Lewis, G. (2000). The reluctance to seek care for neurotic disorders. *Journal of Mental Health*, 9, 319–327.

Mental Health Foundation. (2002). *Taken seriously: The Somerset spirituality project*. London: Mental Health Foundation.

Mesquita, B. (2001). Emotions in collectivist and individualist contexts. *Journal of Personality and Social Psychology*, 80, 68–74.

Meyer, B. (2004). Christianity in Africa: From African independent to pentecostal-charismatic churches. *Annual Review of Anthropology*, 33, 447–474.

Minas, H., & Cohen, A. (2007). Why focus on Mental Health Systems? *International Journal of Mental Health Systems*, 1(1), 1–10.

Minas, H., & Diatri, H. (2008). Pasung: Physical restraint and confinement of the mentally ill in the community. *International Journal of Mental Health Systems*, 2(1), 1–5.

Mino, Y., Yasuda, N., Tsuda, T., & Shimodera, S. (2001). Effects of a one-hour educational program on medical students' attitudes to mental illness. *Psychiatry and Clinical Neurosciences*, 55(5), 501–507.

Mino, Y., Kodera, R., & Bebbington, P. A. (1990). Comparative study of psychiatric services in Japan and England. *British Journal of Psychiatry*, 157, 416–420.

Mitchell, P., Malak, A., & Small, D. (1998). Bilingual professionals in community mental health services. *Australian and New Zealand Journal of Psychiatry*, 32, 424–439.

Miville, M. L., & Constantine, M. G. (2007). Cultural values, counseling stigma, and intentions to seek counseling among Asian American college women. *Counseling and Values*, 52, 2–11.

Mkize, L. P., & Uys, L. R. (2004). Pathways to mental health care in KwaZulu-Natal. *Curationis*, 27(3), 62–71.

Modrow, J. (2003). *How to become a schizophrenic: The case against biological psychiatry*. Lincoln, Nebraska: The Writers Club Press.

Moldovan, V. (2007). Attitudes of mental health workers toward community integration of the persons with serious and persistent mental illness. *American Journal of Psychiatric Rehabilitation*, 10(1), 19–30.

Moller-Leimkuhler, A. M. (2002). Barriers to help-seeking by men: A review of sociocultural and clinical literature with particular reference to depression. *Journal of Affective Disorders*, 71, 1–9.

Monahan, J. (2000). Clinical and actuarial predictions of violence. In D. Faigman, D. Kaye, M. Saks, & J. Sanders (Eds.), *Modern scientific evidence: The law and science of expert testimony* (Vol. 1, pp. 300–218). St. Paul MN: West Publishing Company.

Monteiro, V. B. M., Dos Santos, J. Q., & Martin, D. (2006). Patients' relatives delayed help seeking after a first psychotic episode. *Revista Brasileira de Psiquiatria*, 28, 104–110.

Monteith, M. J. (1996). Affective reactions to prejudice-related discrepant responses: The impact of standard salience. *Personality and Social Psychology Bulletin*, 22, 48–59.

Morgan, C., Mallett, R., Hutchinson G., Jenkins, R., Khandelwal, S., Levav, I., ... Whiteford, H. (2005). Pathways to care and ethnicity. 1: Sample characteristics and compulsory admission. Report from the AESOP study. *British Journal of Psychiatry*, 186, 281–289.

Morris, E., Hippman, C., Murray, G., Michalak, E.E., Boyd, J.E., Livingston, J., ... Austin, J. (2018). Self-Stigma in relatives of people with mental illness scale: Development and validation. *The British Journal of Psychiatry*, 212(3), 169–174.

Mosaku, K. S., & Wallymahmed, A. H. (2017). Attitudes of primary care health workers towards mental health patients: A cross-sectional study in Osun State, Nigeria. *Community Mental Health Journal*, 53(2), 176–182.

Muga, F. A., & Jenkins, R. (2008). Public perceptions, explanatory models and service utilization regarding mental illness and mental health care in Kenya. *Social Psychiatry Psychiatric Epidemiology*, 43, 469–476.

Muirhead, J., & Tilley, J. (1995). Scratching the surface: Mental health training for rural health workers. *Australian and New Zealand Journal of Mental Health Nursing*, 4(2), 95–98.

Mulatu, M. S. (1999). Perceptions of mental and physical illnesses in northwestern Ethiopia: Causes, treatments, and attitudes. *Journal of health psychology*, 4(4), 531–549.

Murali, V., & Oyebode, F. (2004). Poverty, social inequality and mental health. *Advances in Psychiatric Treatment*, 10(3), 216–224.

Murthy, R. S. (2001, August 14). Lessons from Erwadi. Retrieved from http://www.hindu.com/thehindu/2001/08/14/stories/05142524.htm.

Mukherjee, R., Fialho, A., Wijetunge, A., Chesinski, K., & Surgenor, T. (2002). The stigmatization of psychiatric illness: The attitudes of medical students and doctors in a London teaching hospital. *Psychiatric Bulletin*, 26, 178–181.

Naeem, F., Ayub, M., Javid, Z., Irfan, M., Haral, F., & Kingdon, D. (2006). Stigma and psychiatric illness. A survey of attitude of medical students and doctors in Lahore, Pakistan. *Journal of Ayub Medical College, Abbottabad*, 18(3), 46–49.

National Institute for Mental Health in England. (2003). *Inside outside: Improving mental health services for black and minority ethnic communities in England.* London: Department of Health.

Ndetei, D. M., Khasakhala, L. I., Mutiso, V., & Mbwayo, A. W. (2011). Knowledge, attitude and practice (KAP) of mental illness among staff in general medical facilities in Kenya: Practice and policy implications. *African Journal of Psychiatry*, 14, 225–235.

Needham, I., Abderhalden, C., Dassen, T., Haug, H. J., & Fischer, J. E. (2002). Coercive procedures and facilities in Swiss psychiatry. *Swiss Medical Weekly*, 132, 253–258.

Neil, H., & Penny, N. H., OTR/L (2002). Longitudinal study of student attitudes toward people with mental illness. *Occupational Therapy in Mental Health*, 17(2), 49–80.

Neto, F. (2002). Loneliness and acculturation among adolescents from immigrant families in Portugal. *Journal of Applied Social Psychology*, 32, 630–647.

Ngui, E. M., Khasakhala, L., Ndetei, D., & Roberts, L. W. (2010). Mental disorders, health inequalities and ethics: A global perspective. *International Review of Psychiatry*, 22(3), 235–244.

Nichter, M. (1981). Idioms of distress, alternatives in the expression of psychosocial distress: A case study from South India. *Culture, Medicine and Psychiatry*, 5(4), 379–408.

Nickerson, K. J., Helms, J. E., & Terrell, F. (1994). Cultural mistrust, opinions about mental illness and black students' attitudes toward seeking psychological help from white counselors. *Journal of Counseling Psychology*, 41(3), 378–385.

Nicolaidis, C., Timmons, V., Thomas, M. J., Waters, A. S., Wahab, S., Mejia, A., & Mitchell, S. R. (2010). "You don't go tell White people nothing": African-American women's perspectives on the influence of violence and race on depression and depression care. *American Journal of Public Health*, 100(8), 1470–1476.

Nina, A. (2009). International students' awareness and use of counseling services. *McNair Scholars Research Journal*, 5, 29–33.

Njoku, L. (2015, September 6). Sad saga of Enugu's unstable psychiatric hospital. *The Guardian Newspaper*. Retrieved from https://guardian.ng/sunday-magazine/sad-saga-of-enugus-unstable-psychiatric-hospital/.

Nsereko, J. R., Kizza, D., Kigozi, F., Ssebunnya, J., Ndyanabangi, S., Flisher, A. J., ... MHaPP Research Programme Consortium (2011). Stakeholder's perceptions of help-seeking behaviour among people with mental health problems in Uganda. *International Journal of Mental Health Systems*, 5, 5–5.

Nwoko, K. C. (2009). Traditional psychiatric healing in Igbo land, Southeastern Nigeria. *African Journal of History and Culture*, 1(2), 036–043.

Nwokocha, F. I. (2005). *Childrearing practices and communication style of African immigrants and their American-born elementary–age children.* (Doctoral thesis, California State University, Sacramento).

Nwokocha, F. I. (2010). *West African immigrants in Northern California and their attitudes toward seeking Mental Health Services.* (Masters thesis). California State University, Sacramento.

Nyagua, J. Q., & Harris, A. J. (2007). West African refugee health in rural Australia: Complex cultural factors that influence mental health. *African Journal of History and Culture*, 1(2), 36–43.

Nzewi, N. E. (1989). Cultural factors in the classification of Psychopathology in Nigeria. In K. Peltzer and P. O. Ebigbo (Eds.), *Clinical Psychology in Africa* (pp. 208–216). Enugu: Chuka Printing Company Ltd.

Obioha, E. E., & Molale, M. G. (2011). Functioning and challenges of Primary Health Care (PHC) Program in Roma Valley, Lesotho. *Ethno-Medicine*, 5(2), 73–88.

Odejide, A. O., & Olatawura, M. O. (1979). A survey of community attitudes to the concept and treatment of mental illness in Ibadan, Nigeria. *Nigerian Medical Journey*, 9, 343–347.

Odejide, O. A., Oyewunmi, K. L., & Ohaeri, J. U. (1989). Psychiatry in Africa: An overview. *American Journal of Psychiatry*, 146, 708–716.

Oderinde, K. O., Dada, M. U., Kundi, B. M., Benjamin, T. A., Kudale, A. H., ... Abubakar, U. M. (2018). Non-mental health workers' attitudes and perceptions towards people with mental illness in a tertiary health facility in Damaturu, North East Nigeria. *American Journal of Psychiatry and Neuroscience*, 6(2), 46–50.

Odinka, P. C., Oche, M., Ndukuba, A. C., Muomah, R. C., Osika, M. U., Bakare, M. O., ... Uwakwe, R. (2014). The Socio-demographic characteristics and patterns of help-seeking among patients with schizophrenia in south-east Nigeria. *Journal of Health Care for the Poor and Underserved*, 25(1), 180–191.

Office of National Statistics. (1995). *Labour Force Survey*. London: Office of National Statistics.

Ogborn, A. C. (1995). Characteristics of youth and young adults seeking residential treatment for substance use problems: An exploratory study. *Addictive Behavior*, 20(5), 675–678.

Ogunsemi, O. O., Odusan, O., & Olatawura, M. O. (2008). Stigmatising attitude of medical students towards a psychiatry label. *Annals of general psychiatry*, 7(1), 15.

Ogrodniczuk, J. S., Joyce, A. S., & Piper, W. E. (2005). Strategies for reducing patient-initiated premature termination of psychotherapy. *Harvard Review of Psychiatry*, 13(2), 57–70.

Ogunlesi, A. O., & Adelekan, M. L. (1988). Nigerian primary health care workers: A pilot survey on attitude to mental health. *Psychiatric Bulletin*, 12, 441–443.

Ohaeri, J. U. (2001). Caregiver burden and psychotic patient's perception of social support in a Nigerian setting. *Social Psychiatry and Psychiatric Epidemiology*, 36(2), 86–93.

Ohaeri, J. U., & Fido, A. A. (2001). The opinion of caregivers on aspects of schizophrenia and major affective disorders in a Nigerian setting. *Social Psychiatry and Psychiatric Epidemiology*, 36(10), 493–499.

Okafor, E. B. (2009). *The relation between demographic factors and attitudes about seeking professional counseling among adult Nigeria living in the United States.* (Doctoral thesis, University of Akron, Ohio). Retrieved from https://etd.ohiolink.edu/!etd.send_file?accession=akron1258571590&disposition=inline.

Okasha, A. (2007). Message from the WPA president: The WPA global program against stigma and discrimination because of schizophrenia: An update. Retrieved from http://wpanet.org/generalinfo/letter1203.html.

Okhomina, F. O., & Ebie, J. C. (1973). Heat in the head as a psychiatric symptom. In C. C. Adonakoh (Ed.), *Proceedings of the 4th Pan African*

Psychiatric Congress workshop on Neurosis in Africa. Accra: New Times Corporation.

Okpi, A. (2013, August 26). Deporting the Igbo from Lagos insulting – Ohanaeze. *Punch Newspaper Online.* Retrieved from http://www.punchng.com/politics/crossfire/deporting-the-igbo-from-lagos-insulting-ohanaeze/.

Olade, R. A. (1983). Attitudes towards mental illness: Effect of integration of mental health concepts into a post-basic nursing degree programme. *Journal of Advanced Nursing*, 8, 93–97.

Olofsson, B., & Jacobsson, L. (2001). A plea for respect: Involuntarily hospitalized psychiatric patients' narratives about being subjected to coercion. *Journal of Psychiatric and Mental Health Nursing*, 8, 357–366.

Omigbodun, O. O. (2001). A cost-effective model for increasing access to mental health care at the primary care level in Nigeria. *The Journal of Mental Health Policy and Economics*, 4, 133–139.

Onwuejeogwu, M. A. (1986). African indigenous ideology: Communal-individualism. *University of Benin Inaugural Lecture series 24.* Benin City, Nigeria.

Oyegbile, O. (2009). A maddening headache. *Tell*, 22, 47–50.

Ozmen, E., Ogel, K., Aker, T., Sagduyu, A., Tamar, D., & Boratav, C. (2004). Public attitudes to depression in urban Turkey: The influence of perceptions and causal attributions on social distance towards individuals suffering from depression. *Social Psychiatry and Psychiatric Epidemiology*, 39, 1010–1016.

People advocating for change through empowerment (PACE). (1996). *Surviving in thunder bay: An examination of mental mealth issues. Phase 3. Final report of the Action Research Team.* Thunder Bay, Ontario: PACE.

Packer, S., Prendergast, P., Wasylenki, D., Toner, B., & Ali, A. (1994). Psychiatric residents' attitudes toward patients with chronic mental illness. *Hospital and Community Psychiatry*, 45(11), 1117–1121.

Papadopoulos, C., Leavey, G., & Vincent, C. (2002). Factors influencing stigma: A comparison of Greek-Cypriot and English attitudes towards mental illness in north London. *Social Psychiatry & Psychiatric Epidemiology*, 37, 430–434.

Parish, C. (2004). Bennett inquiry finds services scarred by pervasive racism. *Mental Health Practice*, 7(6), 4.

Park, L., Xiao, Z., Worth, J., & Park, J. (2005). Mental health care in China: Recent changes and future challenges. *Harvard Health Policy Review*, 6, 35–45.

Parr, H., & Philo, C. (2003). Rural mental health and social geographies of caring. *Social and Cultural Geography*, 4, 471–488.

Parsons, T. (1951). *The social system.* New York: The Free Press.

Patel, V., Araya, R., Chatterjee, S., Chisholm, D., Cohen, A., De Silva, M., … van Ommeren, M. (2007). Treatment and prevention of mental disorders in low-income and middle-income countries. *Lancet*, 370(9591), 991–1005.

Patel, V., Musara, T., Batau, T., Maramba, P., & Fuyane, S. (1995). Concepts of mental illness and medical pluralism in Harare. *Psychological Medicine*, 25(3), 485–493.

Patel, V., Todd, C., Winston, M., Gwanzura, F., Simunyu, E., Acuda, W., Mann, A. (1997). Common mental disorders in primary care in Harare, Zimbabwe: Associations and risk factors. *The British Journal of Psychiatry*, 171(1), 60–64.

Paterson, B. (2006). Newspaper representations of mental illness and the impact of the reporting of events on social policy: The 'framing' of Isabel Schwarz and Jonathan Zito. *Journal of Psychiatric and Mental Health Nursing*, 13, 294–300.

Pearce, T. O. (1989). Social organisation and psychosocial health. In K. Peltzer & P. O. Ebigbo (Eds.), *Clinical psychology in Africa* (pp. 47–55). Enugu: Chuka Printing Company Ltd.

Peeters, F. P., & Bayer, H. (1999). 'No-show' for initial screening at a community mental health centre: Rate, reasons and further help-seeking. *Social Psychiatry & Psychiatric Epidemiology*, 34, 323–327.

Pelletier, J., Davidson, L., Roelandt, J., & Daumerie, N. (2009). Citizenship and recovery for everyone: A global model of public mental health. *International Journal of Mental Health Promotion*, 11(4), 45–53.

Penn, D. L., Guynan, K., Daily, T., Spaulding, W. D., Garbin, C. P., & Sullivan, M. (1994). Dispelling the stigma of schizophrenia: What sort of information is best? *Schizophrenia Bulletin*, 20, 567–578.

Penny, N. H., Kasar, J., & Sinay, T. (2000). Student attitudes toward persons with mental illness: The influence of course work and level II fieldwork. *The American Journal of Occupational Therapy*, 55, 217–220.

Perlick, D. A., Miklowitz, D. J., Link, B. G., Struening, E., Kaczynski, R., Gonzalez, J. M., ... Rosenheck, R. (2007). Perceived stigma and depression among caregivers of patients with bipolar disorder. *British Journal of Psychiatry*, 190, 535–536.

Perlick, D. A., Rosenheck, R. A., Clarkin, J. F., Sirey, J. A., Salahi, J., Struening, E. L., & Link, B. G. (2001). Stigma as barrier to recovery: Adverse effects of perceived stigma on social adaptation of persons diagnosed with bipolar affective disorder. *Psychiatric Services*, 52,(12), 1627–1632.

Perlick, D. A., Rosenheck, R. A., Clarkin, J. F., Maciejewski, P. K., Sirey, J. A., Struening, E., & Link, B. G. (2004). Impact of family burden and affective response on clinical outcome among patients with bipolar disorder. *Psychiatric Services*, 55, 1029–1035.

Petersen, I., Ssebunnya, J., Bhana, A., & Baillie, K. (2011). Lessons from case studies of integrating mental health into primary health care in South Africa and Uganda. *International Journal of Mental Health Systems*, 5(1), 8–8.

Petty, R. E. (1995). Attitude change. In A. Tesser (Ed.), *Advanced social psychology* (pp. 195–249). New York: McGraw-Hill.

Pfeifer, S. (1994). Belief in demons and exorcism in psychiatric patients in Switzerland. *British Journal of Medical Psychology*, 67(3), 247–258.

Phan, T. (2000). Investigating the use of services for Vietnamese with mental illness. *Journal of Community Health*, 25, 411–425.

Phelan, J., Bromet, E., & Link, B. (1998). Psychiatric illness and family stigma. *Schizophrenia Bulletin*, 24, 115–126.

Phelan, J. C., Link, B. G., Stueve, A., & Pescosolido, B. A. (2000). Public conceptions of mental illness in 1950 and 1996: What is mental illness and is it to be feared? *Journal of Health and Social Behavior*, 41, 188–207.

Philo, G. (1996). *Media and mental distress*. London: Longman.

Pilgrim, D. (2009). *Key concepts in mental health*. London: Sage.

Pinel, E. C. (1999). Stigma consciousness: The psychological legacy of social stereotypes. *Journal of Personality and Social Psychology*, 76, 114–128.

Pinfold, V., Stuart, H., Thornicroft, G., & Arboleda-Florez, J. (2005). Working with young people: The impact of mental health awareness programmes in schools in the UK and Canada. *World Psychiatry: Official Journal of the World Psychiatric Association (WPA)*, 4, 48–52.

Pinfold, V., Toulmin, H., Thornicroft, G., Huxley, P., Farmer, P., & Graham, T. (2003). Reducing psychiatric stigma and discrimination: Evaluation of educational intervention in UK secondary schools. *British Journal of Psychiatry*, 182, 342–346.

Pinto-Foltz, M. D., & Logsdon, M. C. (2009). Reducing stigma related to mental disorders: Initiatives, interventions, and recommendations for nursing. *Archives of Psychiatric Nursing*, 23(1), 32–40.

Pitre, N., Stewart, S., Adams, S., Bedard, T., & Landry, S. (2007). The use of puppets with elementary school children in reducing stigmatizing attitudes towards mental illness. *Journal of Mental Health*, 16(3), 415–429.

Price, E. G., Beach, M. C., Gary, T. L., Robinson, K. A., Gozu, A., Palacio, A., ... Cooper, L. A. (2005). A systematic review of the methodological rigor of studies evaluating cultural competence training of health professionals. *Academic Medicine*, 80, 578–586.

Putman, S. (2008). Mental illness: Diagnostic title or derogatory term? (Attitudes towards mental illness) Developing a learning resource for use within a clinical call centre. A systematic literature review on attitudes towards mental illness. *Journal of Psychiatric and Mental Health Nursing*, 15, 684–693.

Rahman, A., Mubbashar, M. H., Gater, R., & Goldberg, D. (1998). Randomised trial of impact of school mental-health programme in rural Rawalpindi, Pakistan. *Lance*, 352, 1022–1025.

Randhawa, G., & Stein, S. (2007). An exploratory study examining attitudes toward mental health and mental health services among young South Asians in the United Kingdom. *Journal of Muslim Mental Health*, 2(1), 21–37.

Ralph, R. O., & Corrigan, P. W. (2005). *Recovery in mental illness: Broadening our understanding of wellness*. Washington, DC: American Psychological Association.

Ranguram, R., & Weiss, M. (2004). Stigma and somatisation. *The British Journal of Psychiatry*, 185, 174.

Rao, H., Mahadevappa, H., Pillay, P., Sessay, M., Abraham, A., & Luty, J. (2009). A study of stigmatized attitudes towards people with mental health problems among health professionals. *Journal of Psychiatric and Mental Health Nursing*, 16(3), 279–284.

Raymond, C. (1991). Jails reported to be turning into hospitals for the mentally ill. *Chronicle of Higher Education*, 38(15), A16.

Read, J. (2007). Why promoting biological ideology increases prejudice against people labelled "schizophrenic". *Australian Psychologist*, 42, 118–128.

Read, J., & Baker, S. (1996). *Not just sticks and stones: A survey of the stigma, taboos and discrimination experienced by people with mental health problems*. London: Mind.

Reed, F., & Fitzgerald, L. (2005). The mixed attitudes of nurse's to caring for people with mental illness in a rural general hospital. *International Journal of Mental Health Nursing*, 14, 249–257.

Regier, D. A., Hirschfield, R. M., Goodwin, F. K., Burke Jr., J. D., Lazar, J. B., & Judd, L. L. (1988). The NMH depression awareness, recognition and treatment programme: Structure, aims and scientific basis. *American Journal of Psychiatry*, 145, 1351–1357.

Regier, D. A., Narrow, W. E., Rae, S., Manderscheid, W., Locke, Z., & Goodwin, K. (1993). The de facto US mental and addictive disorders service system: Epidemiologic catchment area prospective 1-year prevalence rates of disorders and services. *Archives of General Psychiatry*, 50, 85–94.

Reid, Y., Johnson, S., Bebbington, P., Kuipers, E., Scott, H., & Thornicroft, G. (2001). The longer term outcomes of community care: A 12 year follow-up of the Camberwell High Contact Survey. *Psychological Medicine*, 31, 351–359.

Repper, J., Sayce, L., Strong, S., Willmot, J., & Haines, M. (1997). *Tall stories from the backyard: A survey of 'NIMBY' opposition to community mental health facilities, experienced by key service providers in England and Wales.* London: Mind.

Richmond, I. C., & Foster, J. H. (2003). Negative attitudes towards people with co-morbid mental health and substance misuse problems: An investigation of mental health professionals. *Journal of Mental Health*, 12(4), 393–403.

Rickwood, D. J., & Braithwaite, V. A. (1994). Social-psychological factors affecting help-seeking for emotional problems. *Social Science and Medicine*, 39, 563–572.

Rickwood, D., Deane, F., & Wilson, C. (2007). When and how do young people seek professional help for mental health problems? *Medical Journal of Australia*, 187(7), 35–39.

Rickwood, D., Deane, F., Wilson, C., & Ciarrochi, J. (2005). Young people's help-seeking for mental health problems. *Australian e-Journal for the Advancement of Mental Health*, 4(3), 218–251.

Ritchie, H., & Roser, M. (2018, April). Mental Health. Retrieved from https://ourworldindata.org/mental-health.

Ritsher, J. B., & Phelan, J. C. (2004). Internalized stigma predicts erosion of morale among psychiatric outpatients. *Psychiatry Research*, 129, 257–265.

Roberts, H. (2001). A way forward for mental health care in Ghana? *Lancet*, 357, 1859.

Robertson, J. M., & Fitzgerald, L. F. (1992). Overcoming the masculine mystique: Alternative forms of assistance among men who avoid counselling. *Journal of Critical Psychology, Counseling and Psychotherapy*, 39, 240–249.

Roe, D., Swarbrick, M. (2007). A recovery oriented approach to psychiatric medication: Guidelines for nurses. *Journal of Psychosocial Nursing*, 45(2), 30–35.

Rogers, A., & Pilgrim, D. (2010). *A sociology of mental health and illness*. Milton Keynes, UK: Open University Press.

Rogler, L. H., & Hollingshead, A. B. (1985). *Trapped: Puerto Rican families and Schizophrenia*. Maplewood, NJ: Waterfront Press.

Rogler, L. H., & Cortes, D. E. (1993). Help-seeking pathways: A unifying concept in mental health care. *American Journal of Psychiatry*, 150, 554–561.

Ronzoni, P., Dogra, N., Omigbodun, O., Bella,T., & Atitola, O. (2010). Stigmatization of mental illness among Nigerian schoolchildren. *International Journal of Social Psychiatry*, 56, 507–514.

Rose, D., Thornicroft G., Pinfold V., & Kassam, A. (2007). 250 ways to label people with mental illness. *BMC Health Services Research*, 7, 97.

Rose, E. D. (2010). *Beliefs about mental illness and attitudes towards seeking help: A study of British Jewry*. (Doctoral thesis, University of Hertfordshire, UK). Retrieved from https://uhra.herts.ac.uk/handle/2299/4810.

Rosen, A., Walter, G., Casey, D., & Hocking, B. (2000). Combating psychiatric stigma: An overview of contemporary initiatives. *Australasian Psychiatry*, 8, 19–26.

Rosenhan, D. L. (1973). On being sane in insane places. *Science*, 179(4070), 250–258.

Rost, K., Smith, R., & Taylor, J. L. (1993). Rural-urban differences in stigma and the use of care for depressive disorders. *Journal of Rural Health*, 9, 57–62.

Rüsch, N., Angermeyer, M. C., & Corrigan, P. W. (2005). Mental illness stigma: Concepts, consequences, and initiatives to reduce stigma. *European Psychiatry*, 20, 529–539.

Rüsch, N., Corrigan, P. W., Wassel, A., Michaels, P., Larson, J. E., Olschewski, M., ... Batia, K. (2009). Self-stigma, group identification, perceived legitimacy of discrimination and mental health service use. *British Journal of Psychiatry*, 195(6), 551–552.

Rüsch, N., Evans-Lacko, S. E., Henderson, C., Flach, C., & Thornicroft, G. (2011). Knowledge and attitudes as predictors of intentions to seek help for and disclose a mental illness. *Psychiatric Services*, 62, 675–678.

Russell, J., Thomson, G., & Rosenthal, D. (2008). International student use of university health and counselling services. *Higher Education*, 56, 59–75.

Ryder, A., Bean, G., & Dion, K. (2000). Caregiver responses to symptoms of first-episode psychosis: A comparative study of Chinese and Euro-Canadian families. *Transcultural Psychiatry*, 37(2), 255–265.

Sadock, B. J., & Sadock, V. A. (2007). *Synopsis of psychiatry*. Baltimore: Lippincott Williams and Wilkins.

Sanchez, F., & Gaw, A. (2007). Mental health care of Filipino Americans. *Psychiatric Services*, 58, 810–815.

Sartorius, N. (1998). Stigma: What can psychiatrists do about it? *The Lancet*, 9133(352), 1058–1059.

Sartorius, N. (2002). Iatrogenic stigma of mental illness. *British Medical Journal*, 324, 1470–1471.

Sartorius, N., Gaebel, W., Cleveland, H. R., Stuart, H., Akiyama, T., Arboleda-Flórez, J., ... Tasman, A. (2010). WPA guidance on how to combat stigmatization of psychiatry and psychiatrists. *World Psychiatry: Official Journal of the World Psychiatric Association (WPA)*, 9, 131–144.

Sartorius, N. (2014). Psychiatry in developed and developing countries. In S. Bloch, S. A. Green, & J. Holman, (Eds.), *Psychiatry: Past, present, and prospect* (pp. 117–132). Oxford: Oxford University Press.

Sayce, L., & Boradman, J. (2003). The Disability Discrimination Act 1995: Implications for psychiatrists. *Advances in Psychiatric Treatment*, 9, 397–404.

Sayre, J. (2000). The patient's diagnosis: Explanatory models of mental illness. *Qualitative Health Research*, 10(1), 71–83.

Scheff, T. J. (1966). *Being mentally ill: A sociological theory*. New York: Aldine.

Schomerus, G., Kenzin, D., Borsche, J., Matschinger, H., & Angermeyer, M. C. (2007). The association of schizophrenia with split personality is not an ubiquitous phenomenon: Results from population studies in Russia and Germany. *Social Psychiatry and Psychiatric Epidemiology*, 42, 780–786.

Schomerus, G., & Angermeyer, M. C. (2008). Stigma and its impact on help-seeking for mental disorders: What do we know? *Epidemiology and Psychiatric Sciences*, 17(1), 31–37.

Schomerus, G., Schwahn, C. C., Holzinger, A. A., Corrigan, P. W., Grabe, H. J., Carta, M. G., & Angermeyer, M. C. (2012). Evolution of public attitudes about mental illness: A systematic review and meta-analysis. *Acta Psychiatrica Scandinavica*, 125, 440–452.

Schulze, B. (2007). Stigma and mental health professionals: A review of the evidence on an intricate relationship. *International Review of Psychiatry*, 19(2), 137–155.

Schulze, B., & Angermeyer, M. C. (2003). Subjective experiences of stigma. A focus group study of schizophrenic patients, their relatives and mental professionals. *Social Science and Medicine*, 56, 299–321.

Schulze, B., Richter-Werling, M., Matschinger, H., & Angermeyer, M. C. (2003). Crazy? So what! Effects of a school project on students' attitudes towards people with schizophrenia. *Acta Psychiatrica Scandinavica*, 107, 142–150.

Scott, E. (2017, July 27). New research reveals people with mental illness are facing a 'locked door' when it comes to getting a job. *The Metro*. Retrieved from https://metro.co.uk/2017/07/27/new-research-reveals-people-with-mental-illness-are-facing-a-locked-door-when-it-comes-to-getting-a-job-6808819/.

Sen, M. (2001). *Death by fire: Sati, dowry death and female infanticide in modern India*. London: Weinfield & Nicolson.

Sevilla-Dedieu, C., Kovess-Masféty, V., Haro, J. M., Fernández, A., Vilagut, G., & Alonso, J. (2010). Seeking help for mental health problems outside the conventional health care system: Results from the european study of the epidemiology of mental disorders (ESEMeD). *Canadian Journal of Psychiatry*, 55(9), 586–597.

Shao, W., Williams, J. W., Lee, S., Badgett, R. G., Aaronson, B., & Cornell, J. E. (1997). Knowledge and attitudes about depression among non-generalists and generalists. *The Journal of Family Practice*, 44, 161–168.

Sharrock, J., & Happell, B. (2000). The role of the consultation-liaison nurse in the general hospital. *Australian Journal of Advanced Nursing*, 18, 34–39.

Shea, M., & Yeh, C. J. (2008). Asian American students' cultural values, stigma, and relational self-construal: Correlates of attitudes toward professional help seeking. *Journal of Mental Health Counselling*, 30, 157–172.

Shibre, T., Negash, A., Kullgren, G., Kebede, D., Alem, A., Fekadu, A., ... Jacobsson, L. (2001). Perception of stigma among family members of individuals with schizophrenia and major affective disorders in rural Ethiopia. *Social Psychiatry and Psychiatric Epidemiology*, 36, 299–303.

Shibre, T., Spangeus, A., Henriksson, L., Negash, A., & Jacobsson, L. (2008). Traditional treatment of mental disorders in rural Ethiopia. *Ethiopian Medical Journal*, 46(1), 87–91.

Shulman, N., & Adams, B. (2002). A comparison of Russian and British attitudes towards mental health problems in the community. *International Journal of Social Psychiatry*, 48, 266–278.

Sigelman, L., & Welch, S. (1993). The contact hypothesis revisited: Black-White interaction and positive racial attitudes. *Social Forces*, 71, 781–795.

Simmie, S., & Nunes, J. (2001). *The last taboo – A survival guide to mental health care in Canada*. Toronto: McClelland & Stewart.

Sirey, J. A., Bruce, M. L., Alexopoulos, G. S., Perlick, D. A., Friedman, S. J., & Meyers, B. S. (2001). Stigma as a barrier to recovery: Perceived stigma and patient-rated severity of illness as predictors of antidepressant drug adherence. *Psychiatric Services*, 52(12), 1615–1620.

Skinner, L. J., Berry, K. K., Griffith, S. E., & Byers, B. (1995). Generalizability and specificity of the stigma associated with the mental illness label: A reconsideration twenty-five years later. *Journal of Community Psychology*, 23, 3–17.

Smith, J. P., Tran, G. Q., & Thompson, R. D. (2008). Can the Theory of Planned Behavior help explain men's psychological help-seeking? Evidence for a mediation effect and clinical implications. *Psychology of Men & Masculinity*, 9(3), 179–192.

Sorketti, E. A., Zuraida, N. Z., & Habil, M. H. (2013). Pathways to mental healthcare in high-income and low-income countries. *International Psychiatry*, 10(2), 45–47.

Sorsdahl, K., Stein, D., & Flisher, A. (2013). Predicting referral practices of traditional healers of their patients with a mental illness: An application of the theory of planned behaviour. *African Journal of Psychiatry*, 16(1), 35–40.

Sorsdahl, K., Stein, D. J., Grimsrud, A., Seedat, S., Flisher, A. J., Williams, D. R., & Myer, L. (2009). Traditional healers in the treatment of common mental disorders in South Africa. *Journal of Nervous and Mental Disease*, 6, 434–441.

Song, L. Y., Chang, L. Y., Shih, C. Y., Lin, C. Y., & Yang, M. J. (2005). Community attitudes towards the mentally ill: The results of a national survey of the Taiwanese population. *International Journal of Social Psychiatry*, 51(2), 162–176.

Sosowsky, L. (1980). Explaining the increased arrest rate among mental patients: A cautionary note. *American Journal of Psychiatry*, 137, 1602–1604.

South African Federation of Mental Health (2011). *Understanding mental illness*. Johannesburg: South African Federation of Mental Health.

Soyka, M. (2000). Substance misuse, psychiatric disorder and violent and disturbed behaviour. *British Journal of Psychiatry*, 176, 345–350.

Spector, R. E. (1996). *Cultural diversity in health & illness*. Stamford, CT: Appleton & Lange.

Spinelli, M. (2004). Maternal infanticide associated with mental illness: Prevention and the promise of saved lives. *The American Journal of Psychiatry*, 161(9), 1548–1577.

Steadman, H. J. (1981). Critically reassessing the accuracy of public perceptions of the dangerousness of the mentally ill. *Journal of Health and Social Behavior*, 22, 310–316.

Steadman, H. J., McCarty, D. W., & Morrissey, J. P. (1989). *The mentally ill in jail: Planning for essential services*. New York: The Guilford Press.

Steel, Z., McDonald, R., Silove, D., Silove, D., Bauman, A., Sandford, P., ... Minas, I. H. (2006). Pathways to the first contact with specialist mental health care. *Australia and New Zealand Journal of Psychiatry*, 40, 347–354.

Stephen, M., & Suryani, L. K. (2000). Shamanism, psychosis and autonomous imagination. *Culture, Medicine and Psychiatry*, 24(1), 5–40.

Stern, G., Cottrell, D., & Holmes, J. (1990). Patterns of attendance of child psychiatry out-patients with special reference to Asian families. *British Journal of Psychiatry*, 156, 384–387.

Stout, P. A., Villegas, J., & Jennings, N. A. (2004). Images of mental illness in the media: Identifying gaps in the research. *Schizophrenia Bulletin*, 30, 543–561.

Stuart, H., & Arboleda-Flórez, J. (2001a). Mental illness and violence: Are the public at risk? *Psychiatric Services*, 52(5), 654–659.

Stuart, H., & Arboleda-Flórez, J. (2001b). Community attitudes towards people with schizophrenia. *Canadian Journal of Psychiatry*, 46, 245–252.

Stuart, H. (2005). Why stigma matters and why it should be beaten. *World Psychiatry: Official Journal of the World Psychiatric Association (WPA)*, 4(51), 6–7.

Stuart, H. (2006). Mental illness and employment discrimination. *Current Opinions in Psychiatry*, 19(5), 522–526.

Suan, L., & Tyler, J. (1990). Mental health values and preference for mental health resources of Japanese-American and Caucasian-American students. *Professional Psychology: Research and Practice*, 21(4), 291–296.

Substance Abuse and Mental Health Services Administration (SAMHSA). (2012). *Results from the 2011 National Survey on Drug Use and Health: Mental Health Findings, NSDUH Series H-45, HHS Publication No. (SMA) 12-4725.* Rockville, MD: SAMHSA.

Sue, S. (1977). Community mental health services to minority groups: Some optimism, some pessimism. *American Psychologist*, 32, 616–624.

Sue, D., Sue, D. W., & Sue, S. (1997). *Understanding abnormal behaviour.* New York: Houghton Mifflin Company.

Suite, D. H., La Bril, R., Primm, A., & Harrison-Ross, P. (2007). Beyond mis-diagnosis, misunderstanding and mistrust: Relevance of the historical perspective in the medical and mental health treatment of people of color. *Journal of the National Medical Association*, 99(8), 879–885.

Swanson, J. W., Swartz, M. S., Essock, S. M., Osher, F. C., Wagner, H. R., Goodman, L. A., … Meador, K. G. (2002). The social-environmental context of violent behavior in persons treated for severe mental illness. *American Journal of Public Health*, 92, 1523–1531.

Swanson, J. W., Swartz, M. S., Van Dorn, R. A., Elbogen, E. B., Wagner, H. R., Rosenheck, R. A., … Lieberman, J. A. (2006). A national study of violent behavior in persons with schizophrenia. *Archives of General Psychiatry*, 63, 490–499.

Tabora, B., & Flaskerud, J. (1997). Mental health beliefs, practices, and knowledge of Chinese American immigrant women. *Issues in Mental Health Nursing*, 18, 173–189.

Takeuchi, D. T., Bui, K. V., & Kim, L. (1993). The referral of minority adolescents to community mental health centers. *Journal of Health and Social Behaviour*, 3(4), 153–164.

Tanaka. G., Inadomi, H., Kikuchi, Y., & Ohta, Y. (2006). Evaluating community attitudes to people with schizophrenia and mental disorders using a case vignette method. *Psychiatry and Clinical Neurosciences*, 59(1), 96–101.

Tanaka, G., Ogawa, T., Inadomi, H., Kikuchi, Y., & Ohta, Y. (2003). Effects of an educational program on public attitudes towards mental illness. *Psychiatry and Clinincal Neurosciences*, 57(6), 595–602.

Tang, Y., Sevigny, R., Mao, P., Jiang, F., & Cai, Z. (2007). Help-seeking behaviors of Chinese patients with schizophrenia admitted to a psychiatric hospital. *Administration and Policy in Mental Health and Mental Health Services Research*, 34, 101–107.

Tata, S. P., & Leong, F. T. L. (1994). Individualism-collectivism, social network orientation, and acculturation as predictors of attitudes towards seeking professional psychological help among Chinese Americans. *Journal of Counselling Psychology*, 41, 280–287.

Temmingh, H. S., & Oosthuizen, P. P. (2008). Pathways to care and treatment delays in first and multi episode psychosis. Findings from a developing country. *Social Psychiatry and Psychiatric Epidemiology*, 43(9), 727–735.

ten Have, M., de Graaf, R., Ormel, J., Vilagut, G., Kovess, V., Alonso, J., & ESEMeD/MHEDEA (2010). Are attitudes towards mental health help-seeking associated with service use? Results from the European study of epidemiology of mental disorders. *Social Psychiatry and Psychiatric Epidemiology*, 45(2), 153–163.

Thara, R., & Srinivasan, T. N. (2000). How stigmatising is schizophrenia in India? *International Journal of Social Psychiatry*, 46, 135–141.

The Mental Health Commission. (1998). *Blueprint for mental health services in New Zealand: How things need to be*. Wellington: The Mental Health Commission.

The Mental Health Foundation of New Zealand. (2003). *Respect costs nothing*. Wellington: The Mental Health Foundation of New Zealand.

Thomas, B. (1995). Caught in the frontline. *Nursing Times*, 91, 38–39.

Thomas, D. K. (2008). *West African immigrants' attitudes toward seeking psychological help*. (Doctoral thesis, Georgia State University). Retrieved from https://scholarworks.gsu.edu/cgi/viewcontent.cgi?article=1028&context=cps_diss.

Thompson, A. H., Stuart, H., Bland, R. C., Arboleda-Florez, J., Warner, R., Dickson, R. A., ... World Psychiatric Association (2002). Attitudes about schizophrenia from the pilot site of the WPA worldwide campaign against the stigma of schizophrenia. *Social Psychiatry and Psychiatric Epidemiology*, 37(10), 475–482.

Thomson, A., & Sylvester, R. (1998). Labour's new lad admits to a bit of culture on the side (interview with Frank Dobson). *Daily Telegraph*, January 17, 4.

Thornicroft, G. (2008). Stigma and discrimination limit access to mental health care. *Epidemiologia Psichiatria Sociale*, 17(1), 14–19.

Thornicroft, G. (2013). Premature death among people with mental illness. *British Medical Journal*, 346, f2969.

Thornicroft, G., & Tansella, M. (2002). Balancing community-based and hospital-based mental health care. *World Psychiatry: Official Journal of the World Psychiatric Association (WPA)*, 1(2), 84–90.

Thornton, J. A., & Wahl, O. F. (1996). Impact of a newspaper article on attitudes toward mental illness. *Journal of Community Psychology*, 24, 17–25.

Tilak, J. G. (2002). Education and poverty. *Journal of Human Development*, 3, 2.

Tobin, M. (2000). Developing mental health rehabilitation services in a culturally appropriate context: An action research project involving Arabic speaking clients. *Australian Health Review*, 23, 177–178.

Tófoli, L. F., Andrade, L. H., & Fortes, S. (2011). Somatization in Latin

America: A review on the classification of somatoform disorders, functional syndromes, and medically unexplained symptoms. *Revista Brasileira de Psiquiatria*, 33(1), s59–s80.

Tomcsanyi, T. (2000). Mental health promotion through the dialogue of different philosophies and professions: An interdisciplinary training in mental health. *Mental Health, Religion and Culture*, 2, 143–156.

Torrey, E. F. (1994). Violent behaviour by individuals with serious mental illness. *Hospital and Community Psychiatry*, 45, 653–662.

Torrey, E. F. (1995). *Surviving schizophrenia: A manual for families, consumers and providers*. New York: Harper and Row.

Triandis, H. C. (1989). Cross-cultural studies in individualism and collectivism. In: J. J. German (Ed.), *Nebraska symposium on motivation: Cross-cultural perspectives* (Vol. 37, pp. 41–133). Lincoln: University of Nebraska Press.

Tylee, A. (1999). Training the whole primary care team. In: M. Tansella & G. Thornicroft (Eds.), *Common mental disorders in primary care* (pp. 123–137). London: Routledge.

Tzahr-Rubin, D. (2003). People's willingness to ask for help in time of trouble. *Haifa Forum for Social Work*, 1, 68–93.

Ukpong, D. I., & Abasiubong, F. (2010). Stigmatising attitude towards the mentally ill: A survey in a Nigerian university teaching hospital. *South African Journal of Psychiatry*, 16(2), 56–60.

U.S. Department of Health and Human Services. (1999). *Mental health: A report of the Surgeon General*. Washington, DC: U.S. Department of Health and Human Services.

U.S. Department of Health and Human Services. (2001). *Mental health: A report of the Surgeon General*. Rockville, MD: U.S. Department of Health and Human Services.

UN Permanent Forum on Indigenous Issues. (2014, October 17). History and mandate of the permanent forum. Retrieved from https://www.un.org/development/desa/indigenouspeoples/about-us/permanent-forum-on-indigenou s-issues.html.

UNESCO Institute for Statistics. (2009). Information sheet No. 1: Analysis of the UIS international survey on feature films statistics. Retrieved from http://uis.unesco.org/sites/default/files/documents/analysis-of-the-uis-international-surve y-on-feature-film-statistics-en_0.pdf.

UNESCO Institute for Statistics. (2011). Gross enrolment ratio by level of education. Retrieved from http://data.uis.unesco.org/index.aspx?queryid=142.

UNICEF. (1988). *The Bamako initiative recommendations to the executive board for programme co-ordination 1989–1993*. New York: Bamako Initiative Monitoring Unit, UNICEF.

Uwakwe, R. (2007). The views of some selected Nigerians about mental disorders. *The Nigerian Postgraduate Medical Journal*, 14, 319–324.

Uzochukwu, B. S. C., & Onwujekwe, O. E. (2004). Socio-economic differences and health seeking behaviour for the diagnosis and treatment of malaria: A case study of four local government areas operating the Bamako initiative programme in south-east Nigeria. *International Journal for Equity in Health*, 3(1), 6.

Vaillant, G. E. (2012). Positive mental health: Is there a cross-cultural definition? *World Psychiatry: Official Journal of the World Psychiatric Association (WPA)*, 11, 93–99.

van Boekel, L. C., Brouwers, E. P., van Weeghel, J., & Garretsen, H. F. (2013). Stigma among health professionals towards patients with substance use disorders and its consequences for healthcare delivery: Systematic review. *Drug and Alcohol Dependence*, 131(1), 23–35.

van der Sanden, R. L., Bos, A. E., Stutterheim, S. E., Pryor, J. B., & Kok, G. (2013). Experiences of stigma by association among family members of people with mental illness. *Rehabilitation Psychology*, 58, 73–80.

van't Veer J. T., Kraan, H. F., Drosseart, S. H., & Modde, J. M. (2006). Determinants that shape public attitudes towards the mentally ill: A Dutch public study. *Social Psychiatry Psychiatric Epidemiolology*, 41, 310–317.

Vaughn, L. M., & Holloway, M. (2009). West African immigrant families from Mauritania and Senegal in Cincinnati: A cultural primer on children's health. *Journal of Community Health*, 35(1), 27–35.

Ventevogel, P. (2014). Integration of mental health into primary health care in low-income countries: Avoiding medicalization. *International Review of Psychiatry*, 26(6), 669–679.

Vera, M., Alegria, M., Freeman, D. H., Robles, R., Pescosolido, B., & Pena, M. (1998). Help seeking for mental health care among poor Puerto Ricans: Problem recognition, service use, and type of provider. *Medical Care*, 36, 1047–1056.

Vigo, A., Thornicroft, G., & Atun, R. (2016). Estimating the true global burden of mental illness. *The Lancet*, 3(2), 171–178.

Vogel, D. L., Wade, N. G., & Hackler, A. H. (2007). Perceived public stigma and the willingness to seek counseling: The mediating roles of self-stigma and attitudes toward counseling. *Journal of Counseling Psychology*, 54, 40–50.

Vogel, D. L., & Wade, N. G. (2009). Stigma and help-seeking. *The Psychologist*, 22, 20–23.

Vos, T., Flaxman, A. D., Naghavi, M., Lozano, R., Michaud, C., Ezzati, M., ... Memish, Z. A. (2012). Years lived with disability (YLDs) for 1160 sequelae of 289 diseases and injuries 1990-2010: A systematic analysis for the Global Burden of Disease Study 2010. *Lancet*, 380, 2163–2196.

Wahl, O. F. (1992). Mass media images of mental illness: A review of the literature. *Journal of Community Psychology*, 20, 343–352.

Wahl, O. F., & Harman, C. R. (1989). Family views of stigma. *Schizophrenia Bulletin*, 15(1), 131–139.

Wahl, O. F. (1995). *Media madness: Public images of mental illness*. New Brunswick, NJ: Rutgers University Press.

Wahl, O. F. (1999). Mental health consumers' experience of stigma. *Schizophrenia Bulletin*, 25, 467–478.

Wahl, O., & Aroesty-Cohen, E. (2010). Attitudes of mental health professionals about mental illness: A review of the recent literature. *Journal of Community Psychology*, 38(1), 49–62.

Waldman, S. (2019). *Sacred Liberty: America's long, bloody, and ongoing struggle for religious freedom*. New York: HarperOne.

Wallach, H. S. (2004). Changes in attitudes towards mental illness following exposure. *Community Mental Health Journal*, 40(3), 235–248.

Walters, P. B. (2001). Educational access and the state: Historical continuities and discontinuities in racial inequality in American education. *Sociology of education (extra issue)*, 74(4), 35–49.

Wang, P. S., Berglund, P. A., Olfson, M., & Kessler, R. C. (2004). Delays in initial treatment contact after first onset of a mental disorder. *Health Services Research*, 39(2), 393–415.

Wang, P. S., Demler, O., & Kessler, R. C. (2002). Adequacy of treatment for serious mental illness in the United States. *American Journal of Public Health*, 92, 92–98.

Wang, P. S., Guilar-Gaxiola, S., Alonso, J., Angermeyer, M. C., Borges, G., ... Wells, J. E. (2007). Use of mental health services for anxiety, mood, and substance disorders in 17 countries in the WHO world mental health surveys. *Lancet*, 370(9590), 841–850.

Ware, J. E. Jr., Manning, W. G. Jr., Duan, N., Wells, K. P., & Newhouse, J. P. (1984). Health status and the use of outpatient mental health services. *American Psychologist*, 39(10), 1090–1100.

Warner, L. (2002). *Out at work: A survey of the experiences of people with mental health problems within the workplace.* London: The Mental Health Foundation.

Watson, A. C., Corrigan, P. W., & Ottati, V. (2004). Police officer attitudes and decisions regarding people with mental illness. *Psychiatric Services*, 55, 49–53.

Watters, E. (2010). *Crazy like us: The globalization of the American psyche.* New York: Free Press.

Weinman, J., Petrie, K. J., Sharpe, N., & Walker, S. (2000). Causal attributions in patients and spouses following a heart attack and subsequent lifestyle changes. *British Journal of Health Psychology*, 5, 263–273.

Wells, J. S., McElwee, C. N. G., & Ryan, D. (2000). "I don't want to be a psychiatric nurse": An exploration of factors inhibiting recruitment to psychiatric nursing in Ireland. *Journal of Psychiatric and Mental Health Nursing*, 7, 79–87.

Weller, L., & Grunes, S. (1988). Does contact with the mentally ill affect nurses' attitudes to mental illness? *British Journal of Medical Psychology*, 61, 277–284.

Wellington, P. (1992). *Mental illness and the Arabic, Turkish and Vietnamese communities.* Carlton, Australia: Australian Bicentennial Multicultural Foundation.

Westerlund, D. (1989). Pluralism and change: A comparative and historical approach to African disease etiologies. In A. Jacobson-Widding & D. Westerlund (Eds.), *Culture, experience, and pluralism: Essays on African ideas of illness and healing* (pp. 177–218). Stockholm, Sweden: Almqvist & Wiksell International.

Whittington, R., & Higgins, L. (2002). More than zero tolerance? Burnout and tolerance for patient aggression amongst mental health nurses in China and the UK. *Acta Psychiatrica Scandinavica*, 106(Suppl. 412), 37–40.

White, R. (2013). Globalisation of mental illness. *The Psychologist*, 26(3), 182–185.

Wilson, C. J., Bignell, B., & Clancy, H. (2003). Building bridges to general practice: A controlled trial of the IDGP GPs in Schools program. *PARC Update (Special Issue: Youth Mental Health)*, 8, 19.

Wolff, G., Pathare S., Craig T., & Leff, J. (1996). Community attitudes to mental illness. *British Journal of Psychiatry*, 168, 183–190.

Women against Rape/Legal Action for Women. (1995). *Dossier: The Crown Prosecution Service and the crime of rape*. London: Women against Rape.

Wong, V. L. (1997). *Relationships among degree of acculturation, opinions about mental illness, selected socio-demographic variables and attitudes toward seeking professional psychological help among Chinese college students*. Austin: University of Texas.

Wong, D. F. K. (2007a). Crucial individuals in the help-seeking pathway of Chinese caregivers of relatives with early psychosis in Hong Kong. *Social Work*, 52, 127–135.

Wong, D. F. K. (2007b). Uncovering sociocultural factors influencing the pathway to care of Chinese caregivers with relatives' suffering from early psychosis in Hong Kong. *Culture, Medicine and Psychiatry* 31, 51–71.

World Health Organization. (1978). *Declaration of Alma-Ata: Adopted at the International Conference on Primary Health Care*. Geneva: WHO.

World Health Organization. (1979). *Schizophrenia: An international follow-up study*. Chichester: John Wiley and Sons.

World Health Organization. (2001a). *World Health Report 2001. Mental health: New understanding, new hope*. Geneva: WHO.

World Health Organization. (2001b). Mental health care in developing countries: A critical appraisal of research findings. *World Health Organisation Technical Report Service*, 698, 5–34.

World Health Organization. (2001c). Stop exclusion, dare to care. Retrieved from https://www.who.int/world-health-day/previous/2001/files/whd2001_dare_to_care_en.pdf.

World Health Organization. (2002). *Traditional medicine strategy 2002–2005*. Geneva: WHO.

World Health Organization. (2008). *Mental health gap action program: Scaling up care for mental, neurological and substance use disorders*. Geneva: WHO.

World Health Organization. (2010). *mhGAP intervention guide for mental, neurological and substance use disorders in non-specialized health settings: Mental health Gap Action Programme (mhGAP)*. Geneva: WHO.

World Health Organization. (2011). *Mental health atlas 2011*. Geneva: WHO.

World Health Organization. (2018). *Mental health atlas 2017*. Geneva: WHO.

World Health Organization. (2020). *Depression fact sheet*. Retrieved November 12, 2020, from www.who.int/news-room/fact-sheets/detail/depression.

World Health Organization and International Consortium of Psychiatric Epidemiology (ICPE). (2000). Cross-national comparisons of mental disorders. *Bulletin of the World Health Organization*, 78, 413–426.

World Psychiatric Association. (2002). Community-based Vs. hospital-based mental health care. *World Psychiatry: Official Journal of the World Psychiatric Association (WPA)*, 1(2), 84–101.

World Psychiatric Association. (2005). *The WPA global programme to reduce stigma and discrimination because of schizophrenia: Schizophrenia - Open the Doors training manual*. New York: World Psychiatric Association.

Wrigley, S., Jackson, H., Judd, F., & Komiti, A. (2005). Role of stigma and attitudes toward help-seeking from a general practitioner for mental health problems in a rural town. *Australian and New Zealand Journal of Psychiatry*, 39, 514–521.

Wu, T., Chang, C., Chen, C., Wang, J., & Lin, C. (2015). Further psychometric evaluation of the self-stigma scale-short: Measurement invariance across mental illness and gender. *PLoS ONE*, 10(2), 1–12.

Yang, L. H. (2007). Application of mental disorder stigma theory to Chinese societies: Synthesis and new directions. *Singapore Medical Journal*, 48, 977–985.

Yoshimura, Y., Bakolis, I., & Henderson, C. (2018). Psychiatric diagnosis and other predictors of experienced and anticipated workplace discrimination and concealment of mental illness among mental health service users in England. *Social Psychiatry and Psychiatric Epidemiology*, 53(10), 1099–1109.

Youssef, J., & Deane, F. P. (2006). Factors influencing mental health help-seeking in Arabic-speaking communities in Sydney, Australia. *Mental Health, Religion and Culture*, 9(1), 43–66.

Yusuf, A. J. (2010). Consequences of untreated severe psychiatric disorders in northern Nigeria. *African Journal of Psychiatry*, 13, 92–94.

Zachrisson, H. D., Rodje, K., & Mykletun, A. (2006). Utilization of health services in relation to mental health problems in adolescents: A population based survey. *BMC Public Health*, 6, 34.

Zartaloudi, A., & Madianos, M. G. (2010). Mental health treatment fearfulness and help-seeking. *Issues in Mental Health Nursing*, 31(10), 662–669.

Zimbardo, P. G., & Leippe, M. (1991). *The psychology of attitude change and social influence*. New York: McGraw-Hill.

Index

aberrant behaviour 5, 90
acculturation 47, 101
advocacy 55–61
aesthetics 23
Afana, A. 52
African immigrants 65, 103
African Initiated Churches (AIC) 110
African-American patients 74, 77, 81
aggression: fear of 23; misdirected 90
AIDS 55, 92
Albanians 83
alcohol abuse 6, 18, 19, 50, 70, 78, 98
Al-Krenawi, A. 35
Alma Ata Declaration of 1978 91
alogia 23
alternative care 99, 102, 109, 110,
   112–13, 113, 115, 117, 118–19
alternative healers 109, 118
American Indians 69
American Psychiatric Association 73
Angel, R. 68, 70
anger 32, 48
Angermeyer, M.C. 69, 114
anticipated stigma 32
antidepressants 37, 102
antipsychotics 37
anti-social behaviours 103
anwansi 73, 110–11
anxiety 17, 31, 32, 35, 67, 69, 71,
   90, 101
Arab American women 35
Arab patients 35
Arab women 65
Arboleda-Flórez, J. 10, 54, 56, 60
Arvaniti, A. 43, 87
Asad, T. 42
Asians 11, 64, 65, 88

Association of Nigerian
   Psychiatrists 32
associative stigma 11–3, 42;
   see also stigma
attention deficit hyperactivity disorder
   (ADHD) 70
attitudes: authoritarian 5, 15, 39, 40,
   43–4, 45, 49, 54, 90; social distance 8,
   13, 16, 17, 18, 24, 28, 36, 39–40, 41,
   43, 45, 46–7, 48, 49, 52–4, 89; social
   restriction/restrictiveness 23, 25, 40,
   43–4, 46, 50, 55; stigmatising 43–7,
   48–51, 48–62, 51–5, 55–61, 62
auditory hallucinations 54
Australasian Psychiatric Stigma
   Group 60
Australia 18, 23, 34, 41, 117
Australia Department of Health and
   Aged Care 59
authoritarian attitudes 5, 15, 39, 40,
   43–4, 45, 49, 54, 90
authoritative diagnosis 73
avolition 23
awareness 55–6; in cultural
   competence 121
Ayurvedic medicine 91

babysitters 39
Bailey, S. 90
Baker, S. 33, 86
Bali 67
Barimah, K.B. 101
barriers to mental health care: culture 101;
   and education 105; gender bias 105;
   ideological 65–80, 100–6; inadequacy of
   services 91–5; instrumental 81–99,

100–6; overview 63–4; socio-demographic correlates 100–6
Bell, J.S. 23
Bello, Eniola 115
Bennett, David 75
biogenetics 17–8, 121
biomedical model 109, 117
biomedical psychiatric care 17–8, 93, 119; and alternative care 99; and Asians 68; and colonial mentality 115; complementary model 117–21; compliance 105; cultural appropriateness of 71–3; Eurocentric 103; inadequacy of services 91; limited information on 106; model 109; pathway to 112–14; perception of 79; regional variations 112; rejection of 11; shift from superstitious beliefs to 51; underutilization 76, 78
biopsychosocial causes 17, 19, 51
bipolar disorder 26, 37, 76, 83
Black, Asian and Minority Ethnic (BAME) groups 64, 75
Black patients 74
blood rituals 116
Blueprint for Mental Health Services (New Zealand) 60
Boerner, H. 83
Bolman, W.M. 71
Boradman, J. 25
braig fag syndrome 71
British Psychological Association 74
Brown, B. 27, 32
Bruno, Frank 21
Byrne, P. 51

Cameron, L. 82
Campinha-Bacote, J. 121
Canada 57
Canadian Mental Health Association 9
cannabis 19
cardiovascular diseases 63
'career' of mental illness 3, 6
care-giving 42
Carillo, J.E. 74
catatonia 23
Catholics 45
Cauce, AM. 66, 81, 82
causal attributions for mental illness 16–9; biogenetic 179; biological 17–8; causal 16; of dangerousness 77; defensive 10; mixed 114; religious 45;

situational 10; supernatural 16, 45, 78, 105, 114; theories 16
causal explanations: biopsychosocial 17; supernatural 16–7
CBS 58
Changing Mind campaign 59
charms 111
Chaucer, Geoffrey 110
Chew-Graham, C. 65
child abuse 35
child health 30
China 42
Christianity 116
Christians 110, 111
Churchill, Winston 42
circulatory diseases 63
Citizens Advice Bureau 26
Clark, L. 101
clinicians 67, 94, 102
cognitive dissonance 13
cognitive individuation 53
cognitive stigma 53
cognitive theory 107
cognitive tolerance 109
Cohen, A. 71
cold-shouldering 10
collectivist cultures 11, 14, 15, 42, 65, 82, 83–4
colonial mentality 115
common mental disorders (CMD) 69
communialism 28, 73
communitarian cultures 11, 12, 15, 28–9, 81, 84, 96
Community Attitudes towards Mental Illness (CAMI) scale 97
community care 20, 28–9, 43, 46
co-morbidity 36, 37, 55
complementary care 98–9, 102, 117–21
conformity 12, 15, 66
consequences of stigma 25–37; burden of disease 32–3; help-seeking impedance 33–5; social exclusion 25–30; structural discrimination 30–2; treatment and recovery impedance 35–7
consumer movements 55
contact 51–5
coping mechanisms 1, 17, 23, 54, 80, 81, 83, 90, 93, 114
Corrigan, P.W. 3, 55, 58
Crawford, P. 27, 32
Crazy like Us 68
Crazy People (movie) 41, 58–9

criminalisation 31
cross-referrals 119
cultivation theory 21–2
cultural appropriateness 71–6
cultural competence 73, 75, 102, 121
culture 1, 14–5, 65; collectivist 11, 14, 15, 42, 65, 82, 83–4; communitarian 11, 12, 15, 28–9, 81, 84, 96; host 101; native 101

deinstitutionalisation 1–2, 25, 28, 29–30, 40
deliverance 110
Delivering Race Equality (DRE) 75
Demler, O. 36
demographics: Asians 11, 64, 65, 88; BAME (Black, Asian and Minority Ethnic groups) 64, 75; Catholics 45; ethnic minorities 47, 64, 68, 72, 73–5, 91, 101, 102–3; Evangelicals 45, 115–16; familiarity with mental illness 43; females 31, 35, 44, 80, 105; general public 8, 40, 42, 45, 46, 69, 79, 86, 103; low education 105–6; low-income countries 64, 106; male 44, 105; middle-income countries 64, 106; nurses 13, 23, 39–40, 45–6, 49, 52, 53, 54, 56, 60, 83, 87, 90, 91, 103; old 8, 43; Protestants 45, 110; students 40, 45, 46, 49–50, 54–5, 65, 67, 69, 71, 76, 79, 103; teachers 25–6, 40, 45, 46, 60, 103, 104; young 43, 80, 101, 103–4
depression 10, 11, 18, 23, 31, 32, 35, 41, 42, 67, 69, 71, 98, 101
Desforges, D.M. 52
desire, in cultural competence 121
Dessoki, H. 44
destitution 121
Determinants of Outcome of Severe Mental Disorder (DOSMeD) 121
developed world 41–3
developing world 38–41
deviance 15, 66
deviation 15
diabolism 116
Diagnostic and Statistical Manual of Mental Disorders (DSM) 115
diagnostic terms 89
difference 15
Dinos, S. 67, 114
Disability Discrimination Act 55

disability-adjusted life-years (DALYs). 63
disabled person 73
discouragement 32
discrimination 3–4, 4, 13, 27, 29, 30–2, 33–4, 36, 38, 53, 54, 55–7, 59, 60, 67, 78, 85, 86, 88, 92, 96
diseases, conceptualisation of 68–70
disorder(s): alcohol abuse 6, 18, 19, 50, 70, 78, 98; anxiety 17, 31, 32, 35, 67, 69, 71, 90, 101; attention deficit hyperactivity disorder (ADHD) 70; bipolar 26, 37, 76, 83; depression 10, 11, 18, 23, 31, 32, 35, 41, 42, 67, 69, 71, 98, 101; post-traumatic stress syndrome (PTSD) 35, 68–9, 119; schizoaffective 114; schizophrenia. See schizophrenia
distress 16, 29, 32, 34, 35, 49, 50, 54, 61, 63, 65, 67, 68, 70, 73, 77, 79, 85, 88, 94, 100, 113, 119
divination 111
diviners 111
divorce 35, 44, 49, 105
doctors 25, 26, 32, 39, 49, 50, 52, 67, 78, 85, 87, 89, 95, 110
Dohrenwend, B.P. 14
Donati, F. 87
Donnelly, P.J. 82
Dow, H.D. 83
drug abuse 18, 41, 50, 51, 90, 101
drug peddlers 93
drug store operators 93
drug vendors 93
Drummond, P.D. 66
Duckworth, K. 20
Dunn 27

Earle, K.A. 69
Eastern Europe 109
education: and help-seeking behaviour 105–6; role in improving stigmatising attitudes 48–51
El Salvador 60
elective office 30
embarrassment 32, 87
emotions 3, 11, 32, 62, 63, 67, 80, 90
employment 26, 40, 50, 84
enchantment 19
encounter, in cultural competence 121
epidemiology: cardiovascular diseases 63; circulatory diseases 63;

disability-adjusted life-years (DALYs). 63; years lived with disability (YLDs) 63
Erase the Stigma campaign 61
Erwadi tragedy 41
Ethiopia 38, 51, 117
ethnic minorities 101; access to mental health services 72, 91, 101; and cultural appropriateness of service 73–5; help-seeking behaviour 102; mental health care utilisation 64; negative attitudes 47; perception of mental health 102–3; suspicion on White-dominated service 68; understanding of mental illness 68
Evangelical Churches 116
Evangelical pastors 115
evidence-based interventions (EBIs) 75
exorcism 111
explanatory models (EMs) 16, 68, 70

faith healers 93, 101, 110–11, 116, 117
families 14; abandonment by 33, 38, 63; financial burden on 93; stigma to 11–2, 14, 35; stress 15, 28–9
family honour 65
family members 3, 11, 12, 13, 15, 29, 30, 36, 38, 39, 41, 66, 81, 82, 83, 105, 114, 118
family relationships 27, 29, 55
fasting 91, 110
fear 8, 10, 11, 12, 19, 21–2, 26, 32, 34, 36, 48, 69, 87–8
Fernando, Gaithri 68
Fitzgerald, L. 87, 90
Foucault, M. 8
free market model 109–11
friendships 27, 118
Fujisawa, D. 98

Gamer, James 58
Gehlot, P.S. 14
gender stereotyping 44, 79, 105
general practitioners 52, 95, 109, 117; discrimination from 88; low therapeutic commitment of 86–7
general public 8, 40, 42, 45, 46, 69, 79, 86, 103
Germany 52, 57, 69
Goffman, Erving 3, 12
Good, G.E. 80

gossips 14, 28, 29, 101
Graham, J.R. 35
Greece 42
gross domestic product (GDP) 92
group identity 12
guilt 32
Gulliver, A. 104
Gureje, O. 38

Hallmark Cards 58
Halloween costumes 42
hallucination 66
Hannah, Daryl 59
Harman, C.R. 20
health insurance 31
health workers 52; attitude of 97; discrimination from 88; distancing behaviour 39–40; negative attitudes of 22–3, 46, 49, 51–2, 85, 87, 88, 89; rejecting attitudes of 37; stigma in practice of 29; stigmatising attitudes 89–90; training of 98
help-seeking behaviour 33–5; gender differences in 105; ideological barriers 65–80; instrumental barriers 81–99; socio-demographic correlates of barriers 100–6; and symptom severity 113; treatment fearfulness 87–8
help-seeking pathway 79, 81, 115
Hifnawy, T.M.S. 44
Hispanic patients 84
HIV/AIDS 55, 92
Hofsess, L. 101
Hollingshead, A.B. 114
holy oils 110
holy water 110
homelessness 27, 29, 50
homicidal madman stereotype 8–9
hospitalisation 11, 12, 15, 23–4, 39, 40, 66, 70
host culture 101
Howells, K. 15
Hsu, G. 83
Hugo, M. 22–3, 117
human capital theory 106
human rights 39, 87
Hungary 120
Hungerfold massacre of 1987 8
hurt 32
Huxley, P. 53
hypnotics 37
hysterical paralysis 73

iatrogenic stigma 85, 90;
  see also stigma
ideological barriers 65–80; and
  acculturation 101; conceptualisation
  of disease 68–70; cultural
  appropriateness of care 71–6; culture
  of self-reliance 79–80; versus
  instrumental barriers 100–6; and
  mental health literacy 76–9; socio-
  demographic correlates 100–6
Igbo people 8–9, 12, 15, 23, 28, 33, 66,
  80, 81–2; *see also* ethnic minorities
Ikwuka, U. 43, 113
illness: perceptions 16; Western models
  of 68
immigrants 7, 67; acculturation 101;
  African 65, 103; Asian 65; from
  collectivist cultures 82; cultural/
  linguistic barriers 68, 75–6;
  identification with native cultures 101
imperialisation of mental health 115
In Our Own Voice programme 58
incantation 111
incarceration 31
incense, burning of 110
India 41, 115
indigenous medicine 91
infant mortality 92
infectious diseases 30
insanity 34, 70
institutional stigmatisation 28
institutionalism 1
instrumental barriers 81–99; awareness
  of available healthcare services
  101–2; and education 105;
  experience of mental health system
  85–90; gender bias 105; versus
  ideological barriers 100–6; service
  inadequacy 91–5; social network
  81–5; socio-demographic
  correlates 100–6
insurance 31, 36, 93
integrated primary care 95–9
internalised stigma 10
International Classification of Diseases
  (ICD) 71, 115
International Pilot Study of
  Schizophrenia (IPSS) 120–1
International Study of Schizophrenia
  (ISoS) 121
inter-personal relationships 27
interventions, evidence-based 75
intimacy 8

isolation 32
Italy 42
izzat 65

Japan 42, 109
Japanese Americans 69
Jorm, A.F. 18
jury duty 30

Kanuri people 13
Kazakhstan 91
Kermode, M. 55
Kessler, R.C. 36
Keynejad, R. 72, 102
kinship 12, 28, 118
knowledge, in cultural competence 121
Komiti, A. 28
koro 71
KwaZulu – Natal, South Africa 113

labelling 5–6, 88–9
Lalani, N. 20
Lambo, T.A. 66
landlords 41
The Last Taboo 11
laws 31
Lesotho 120
Levey, S. 15
life insurance 31
Lin, K.M. 76
Link, B.G. 78
Litwak, E. 118
local government area 95, 97–8
London, C. 20
low education 105–6
low-income countries 64, 106
Lunacy Act 32

Maccoby, E.E. 43, 44
madness 7, 8, 17, 33, 36, 37, 70;
  see also schizophrenia
Makanjuola, V.Y. 17, 19
Malawi 38
Marie Balter Story (movie) 58
marriage 27, 30, 41
mass communication theories 21–2
mass media 19–22
maternal health 30
maternal mortality 92
McVeig, Tracy 115

media, (mis)representation of mental illness in 19–22, 57–8
media portayals 19–22
medical students 50
medications 10, 23, 27, 37, 83, 85, 88, 95, 99, 101, 102, 111, 114, 117
medicine: indigenous 91; mild 37; strong 37; traditional 71, 111, 116; Western 71
Mehta, N. 20
mending face 10
mental disorders: bipolar disorder 26, 37, 76, 83; depression 10, 11, 18, 23, 31, 32, 35, 41, 42, 67, 69, 71, 98, 101; hysterical paralysis 73; psychosis 16, 18, 19, 27, 31, 36, 41, 51, 67, 79, 98, 118; psychotic behaviour 8; psychotic conditions 4, 15, 78
Mental Health Act 20
Mental Health American (MHA) 57–8
Mental Health Awareness Week 55
mental health care: complementary model 117–21; cultural appropriateness of 71–6; inadequacy of services 91–5; integration into primary health care 95–9
mental health education 50–1
Mental Health Gap Action Programme Intervention Guide (mhGAP-IG) 97
mental health indicators, cultural variations in 69
mental health literacy 76–9
mental health staff 87
mental health system, experience of 85–90
mental illness: attitudes towards 1–2; causal explanations for 16–9; diagnosis of 23–4; incidence of 63; labelling 5–6, 69; misconceptualisation of 19–22; misrepresentation of 19–22; nature and symptom presentation of 22–3; portrayal in media 19–22; stigmatisation of 1
mental patients 5, 7, 21, 42, 95
mentally ill 5, 8, 11, 20, 26, 32, 36, 86, 105
mentally illl killers 20
Mexican Americans 68
middle-income countries 64, 106
mild medicine 37
Minas, H. 71

minority groups 53, 71, 72, 73–4, 91, 92, 101, 103; *see also* ethnic minorities
misdirected aggression 90
Mkize, L.P. 37, 77, 84
modified labelling theory 90
Moldovan 25
Moore, Dudley 59
Morocco 38, 44
mortality 16, 101
motor mechanics 23
movies 19–20
Muller, Margaret 20–1
multiple personality 69
Murali, V. 93

Nathawat, S.S. 14
National Alliance on Mental Illness (NAMI) 58
National Co-morbidity Survey 36
National Health Service 26, 28, 75, 102–3, 119
National Mental Health Association 57–8
National Mental Health Council (El Salvador) 60
Ndetei, D.M. 52
negative attitudes 14–8, 19, 22, 38, 40, 41, 42, 48, 54, 68, 85–6, 89, 90; adverse impact of 89; and age 43; demographic correlates 43–7; gender differences in 44; of health workers 22–3, 46, 49, 51–2, 85, 86, 87, 88, 89
negative experiences 88
neighbours 3, 5, 10, 12, 29, 41, 82, 86, 118
Netherlands 18
neuropsychiatric hospitals 95
New Zealand 36, 42, 60
NHS Trust 120
Nigeria 8–9, 13, 16, 17, 19, 25, 31–2, 39–40, 43–4, 48, 66, 69–70, 77, 78, 81–2, 93–4, 96, 100, 112, 116, 118; healthcare spending allocation in 92; psychiatric facilities in 95; psychiatric patients 11
Nigerian Federal Ministry of Health (FMOH) 91
Nigerian University 5
NIMBY (not in my backyard) attitude 28
Nollywood 19, 115

Non-English-Speaking Backgrounds (NESB) 73
no-show 72
nurses 13, 23, 39–40, 49, 52, 53, 54, 56, 60, 83, 87, 90, 91, 103; negative attitudes 45–6; perceived ideological and instrumental barriers 103
Nwokocha, F.I. 67
Nzewi, N.E. 72, 73

occupational therapy 73
Odejide, A.O. 53
Ogborn, A.C. 85, 90
Ogun State 25
Oh, E. 18
Olatawura, M.O. 53
Onwujekwe, O.E. 80
onyeara 8–9
Open the Doors programme 26, 56
Opinion about Mental Illness (OMI) Scale 49
ostracism 1, 7
Oyebode, F. 93

Pakistan 120
Papadopoulos, C. 43
Paramount Pictures 58
The Pardoner's Tale (Chaucer) 110
parenting 30
pastors 115
Patel, V. 113
paternalism 65
pathways to mental healthcare 109–11; biomedical model 109, 117; free market model 109–11; overview 107–8; and social desirability 115; spiritual pathway 110–11; in sub-Saharan Africa 112–16
Pearce, T.O. 14
Penn, D.L. 23, 58
people with disabilities 73
performance failures 14
pervasiveness of stigma: in developed world 41; in developing world 38–41
pharmacies 95
pharmacy students 23
physical illness 37, 38, 67, 78
physical symptoms 67, 68, 94
Pilgrim, D. 26
post-traumatic stress syndrome (PTSD) 35, 68–9, 119

poverty 27, 50, 92, 93–4, 100
prayers 91, 110
predisposing factors 14–24; causal explanations 16–9; culture 14–5; diagnosis of mental illness 24; mental illness conceptualisation/ representation 19–22; nature and symptom presentation of illness 22–3; psychiatric hospitalisation 24
prejudice 1, 3, 10, 13, 19, 22, 33, 34, 47, 52, 56, 70, 89, 92
primary health care 91, 94, 95–9
Primary Health Care Operations Research (PRICOR) 92
primary health care (PHC) 91–3
prognosis, pessimism of 11, 16, 17, 19, 39, 44, 103
Promise (movie) 58
prophesying 110
prostitutes 6
Protestants 45, 110
psychiatric care: cultural appropriateness of 71–6; experience of 85–90; stigmatization in 88
psychiatric facilities 95, 112, 117
psychiatric hospitalisation 11, 12, 15, 23–4, 40, 66, 70
psychiatrists 4; in care pathway 112, 118; inadequacy of 91, 95; indigenous 119; integrated primary care 98; lack of rapport with mental health patients 87; in Nigeria 91; referral to 34; salaries 85–6; stereotypes 13; stigmatising attitudes of 57
psycho killer 20
psychologists, stereotypes 13
psychosis 6, 16, 18, 19, 27, 31, 36, 41, 51, 67, 69, 79, 98, 118
psychotic disorders 7, 19, 25, 63, 69–70, 117
psychotic vagrants 5
public health campaigns 79
public office 39
public stigma 8–10
puerperal psychosis 35
Puerto Rico 114
Punjabis 64

Ranguram, R. 67
rape 31

Read, J. 33, 85
recovery 11, 16, 19, 30, 32, 35–7, 58, 68, 73
reductionist approach 4
Reed, F. 87, 90
referrals 74, 79, 87, 91, 94, 98, 109, 118–19, 121
Regier, D.A. 69
religiosity 44–5
Report on Mental Health 30
Repper, J. 28
Rethink Mental Illness 42
rituals 111, 116
roadside pharmacies 95
Rogler. L.H. 114
Rosenhan, D.L. 5
Rotary International 61
Royal College of Psychiatrists 59
Russell, J. 67
Russia 69

sacramentals 110
Sartorius, N. 85–6, 89
saving face 15
Sayce, L. 25
Scheff, T.J. 4
schizoaffective disorder 114
schizophrenia 76, 93–4, 103; ability to live with 50; in adolescence and young adulthood 103; awareness in patients 76; biological factors 17–8; burden on families 93; concerns of people with 41; in developed world 41–2; and employment 10, 26; fear of 155; labelling 5, 33, 69; long-term social outcomes of 29; low research funding for 30; in newspapers 20; number of people worldwide with 57; paranoid 45; reducing the stigma of 53, 56; shame to families 12; stigmatisation of 4, 15, 22, 27, 38–9; supported education programme for adults with 36; survivor 4; symptom presentation 22–3; and violence 21
Schulze, B. 53
Scott, E. 26
secrets 14, 34, 40, 66
sedatives 37
See Me campaign 20
self-efficacy 32
self-esteem 11, 32
self-loathing 10

self-medication 93
self-reliance 79–80
self-stigma 10–1, 17, 19; *see also* stigma
serious and persistent mental illness (SPMI) 25
sex-role stereotyping 80
shame 12, 15, 34, 65, 66
Sharby, Nancy 83
skill, in cultural competence 121
Skinner, L.J. 6
slumlords 41
social cognitive theory 21–2
social conditioning 47
social conflicts 85
social desirability 115
social distance 8, 13, 16, 17, 18, 24, 28, 36, 39–40, 41, 43, 45, 46–7, 48, 49, 52–4, 89
social exclusion 25–30
social instability 42
social labeling 88–9
social learning theory 54
social networks 81–5, 118
social rejection 101
social reputation 15
social restriction/restrictiveness 23, 25, 40, 43–4, 46, 50, 55
sociocultural differences 72
sociological theories 3
socio-psychological processes of stigma 3–7
soldiers 34–5
somatisation 67, 69
somatoform symptoms 119
sorcery 19
South Africa 94, 117
South African Federation of Mental Health (SAFMH) 34, 61
South African Mental Health Movement (SAMHAM) 61
Soyinka, Wole 110
spirit-based belief 76, 78
spiritual curses 16–7
spiritual healers 93, 101, 119
spiritual pathway 110–11
split personality 69
Sri Lanka 68
stereotypes 8–9, 101
stigma: actor 3; anticipated 32; associative 11–3, 42; audience 3; cognitive 53; components of 3; consequences of 25–37; etymology of 3; iatrogenic 85, 90; pervasiveness of 38–48; predisposing factors 14–24;

process 53; public 8–10; as second illness 32; self-stigma 10–1; sociological theories of 3; socio-psychological processes 3–7; types of 8–13; vicarious 13
stigmatising attitudes 51–5; advocacy 55–61; demographic correlates 43–7; and education 48–51; improving 48–62; multidimensional approach to 62; *see also* negative attitudes
Stop Exclusion, Dare to Care programme 57
strange occurrences 114
strong medicine 37
structural discrimination 30–2
Suan, L. 69
sub-Saharan Africa 16–7, 18, 19, 22, 23, 67, 72, 98, 109–10, 112–16
substance abuse 18, 41, 50, 51, 90, 101
Substance Abuse and Mental Health Service Administration (SAMHSA) 59
suicides 14, 19, 36
supermarkets 42
supernatural causation 11, 16–7, 19, 43, 78, 114, 119
Supported Education Programme (SEP) 36
symptoms: concealment of 10; living in denial of 10, 35; presentation 22–3; somatoform 119

Taijikistan 61
teachers 25–6, 40, 45, 46, 60, 103, 104
Teijlingen, E.R.V. 101
television shows 20
tertiary care 94–5, 96
Tesco 42
therapeutic alliance 70, 73, 87, 119, 121
therapists 64, 70, 72–6, 90, 102, 114
Thoits, P. 68, 70
Thornicroft, G. 118
Thornton, J.A. 22
Time to Change initiative 59, 86
Torrey, E.F. 24
traditional healers 67, 93, 110–11, 116, 117, 118
traditional medicine 71, 111, 116
treatment: fearfulness 87–8; impedance of 35–7
The Trials of Brother Jero (Soyinka) 110
Turkey 52
Turkish population 18
Tyler, J. 69

Uganda 112–13
ultimate stigma 6–7
UN Permanent Forum on Indigenous Issues 118
Unani medicine 91
uninsured 93
Union of Mental Health Support (Taijikistan) 61
United Kingdom 42
urbanisation 93
user fees 95
Uys, L. 37, 77, 84
Uzochukwu, B.S.C. 80

vagrancy 70
vagrants 5, 6, 23, 29, 31, 33, 51, 70
veterans 34–5
vicarious stigma 13
Vietnamese 64
Village Destroyers (movie) 5
violence 8, 20, 21–2, 25, 30, 43, 46, 50, 50–1, 115
voting 30

Wahl, O.F. 20, 22
Wang, P.S. 36
Watson, A.C. 3
Watters, E. 68
Weiss, M. 67
West Africa 71
West African refugees 66
Western medicine 71
Western models of illness 68
Wood, K. 80
Woods, James 58
Woolley, S.R. 83
World Health Organisation (WHO) 27, 56, 57, 91, 96
World Mental Health Day 55
World Psychiatric Association (WPA) 1, 26, 48, 56, 100

years lived with disability (YLDs) 63
Yemenis 11–2
young people: anti-social behaviours 101; help-seeking behaviour 103–4; perceived ideological and instrumental barriers 103; views on mental health 104

Zimbabwe 113

Printed in the United States
by Baker & Taylor Publisher Services